PRAISE FOR
IT'S NOT YOUR FAULT

'Alex Howard has done it again! *It's Not Your Fault* is a book that will benefit everyone, though the reader will feel it was written specifically for them. Alex addresses a complex topic with empathy and understanding while providing tools to navigate the impacts of past traumatic experiences.'

ANDREA NAKAYAMA, FUNCTIONAL MEDICINE NUTRITIONIST, EDUCATOR, AND SPEAKER

'Alex Howard squarely places himself among the giants with *It's Not Your Fault*, where he brings mind-body medicine from an idea to life with heart, stories, and vulnerability. *It's Not Your Fault* is a candid and refreshingly honest journey into the wounds and emotions we do everything to NOT feel and the powerful path through to the freedom we each desire for our future. *It's Not Your Fault* is an essential, practical, and living read for anyone with a human body, emotions, chronic illness, or in the chaos of escaping emotions. I recommend this book to all those seeking healing!'

DR. AIMIE APIGIAN, FOUNDER AND CEO OF TRAUMA ACCELERATED HEALING

'Heartfelt, powerful, and brilliant – this could be the best book on trauma I've ever read. It combines good science on the neuropsychology of trauma, personal stories, and tons of useful methods. Alex Howard provides a new comprehensive framework to move this field forward. Clearly and beautifully written, it carries the reader along quickly, with useful insights, warm encouragement, and practical tools on every page. A gem.'

DR. RICK HANSON, *NEW YORK TIMES* BEST-SELLING AUTHOR
OF *HARDWIRING HAPPINESS* AND *RESILIENT*

IT'S NOT YOUR FAULT

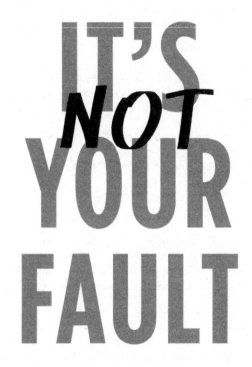

IT'S NOT YOUR FAULT

Why childhood trauma shapes you and how to break free

Alex Howard

HAY HOUSE

Carlsbad, California • New York City
London • Sydney • New Delhi

Published in the United Kingdom by:
Hay House UK Ltd, The Sixth Floor, Watson House, 54 Baker Street
London W1U 7BU
Tel: +44 (0)20 3927 7290; Fax: +44 (0)20 3927 7291; www.hayhouse.co.uk

Published in the United States of America by:
Hay House Inc., PO Box 5100, Carlsbad, CA 92018-5100
Tel: (1) 760 431 7695 or (800) 654 5126; Fax: (1) 760 431 6948 or (800) 650 5115
www.hayhouse.com

Published in Australia by:
Hay House Australia Ltd, 18/36 Ralph St, Alexandria NSW 2015
Tel: (61) 2 9669 4299; Fax: (61) 2 9669 4144; www.hayhouse.com.au

Published in India by:
Hay House Publishers India, Muskaan Complex, Plot No.3, B-2,
Vasant Kunj, New Delhi 110 070
Tel: (91) 11 4176 1620; Fax: (91) 11 4176 1630; www.hayhouse.co.in

A catalogue record for this book is available from the British Library.

Tradepaper ISBN: 978-1-83782-077-1
E-book ISBN: 978-1-83782-079-5
Audiobook ISBN: 978-1-83782-078-8

Printed and bound by CPI Group (UK) Ltd, Croydon CR0 4YY

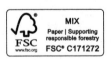

To my two most important teachers:
Sandra Maitri and Prakash Mackay.
I fear I wasn't always an easy student, but I hope
this book shows that your love and patience were
not wasted, and a few things did sink in!

CONTENTS

Part III: The ABCD of Healing in the Real World

A NOTE FROM THE AUTHOR

When writing a book about trauma, one is highly aware of standing on the shoulders of giants, and this is uppermost in my mind because I have the privilege of interviewing many of the pioneers of trauma research for the annual Trauma Super Conference.

My conversations with such experts as Dr. Peter Levine (Somatic Experiencing®), Professor Stephen Porges (Polyvagal Theory), Dr. Gabor Maté (Compassionate Inquiry®), Thomas Hübl (Collective Trauma), and Dr. Arielle Schwartz (Eye Movement Desensitization and Reprocessing, or EMDR, and Therapeutic Yoga), to name just a few, have impacted me significantly.

While planning the content of this book, I had to make some sensitive choices. It was tempting to produce a 'greatest hits' of the extraordinary body of work in this field, but I chose not to for several reasons. Firstly, there are some excellent books and blogs that already do this job well; and secondly, I wanted to create a practical and effective roadmap for change informed by my own personal experience and 20 years in clinical practice.

Given that my psychology-based online RESET Program® is 30 hours in duration, and that my team and I have recorded more than 250 hours of interviews for our Trauma Super Conference series, my challenge in writing this book was to prevent it from becoming overly complex or pulling in too many directions at once. Therefore, may I ask you to assume that the omission of others' ideas and theories is made in full awareness of and respect for their work. And in the spirit of delivering a guide with tools that you can use today to create change in your life and reset the impacts of your trauma.

PART I

Decode Your Trauma

CHAPTER 1
The Wounds That Shape Us

It was a cold, frosty early morning in South Wales and the final day of a week-long retreat in which I was taking part, something I did several times a year to understand myself more deeply. As a successful therapist, I ought to have been in my comfort zone and having the time of my life, but in truth, I was in my own personal hell.

Unable to sleep and needing to move my body, I decided to take a walk to try and clear my head. The silence of the retreat center was palpable as I slipped out the back door and followed one of the routes into the forest behind the building. As I picked up the pace to keep warm, my mind drifted back to the previous day's teachings.

The subject of the retreat was opening to our unprocessed emotions and learning to feel them and heal them. The idea sounded simple, but to me, it felt like a path worse than death. In fact, several years earlier, I'd attended this same retreat and halfway through I'd walked out mid-lecture and driven home, telling myself it just wasn't for me.

At this time, my emotions were far from being a safe place; indeed, I was starting to realize that unconsciously, I'd designed my life in such a way as to avoid feeling them. The problem was it was becoming harder to do so.

My Trauma Healing Journey

In the 18 months prior to the retreat, I'd experienced debilitating panic attacks that had almost consumed my life. During the daytime, I ran the gauntlet of anxiety and fear, but that was nothing compared to nighttime, when I had to face the terror without distractions; at one point, I found myself in one unhealthy relationship after another simply as an alternative to sleeping alone. I'd always been proudly independent, so this situation had only deepened my sense of hopelessness.

The timing of my falling apart couldn't have been more disastrous. At the age of 26 I'd already achieved many of my dreams – after fighting a seven-year battle with myalgic encephalomyelitis, also known as chronic fatigue syndrome (ME/CFS), as a teenager, I'd gone on to make a full recovery and had set up the kind of clinic that I'd longed for when I was ill: one specializing in fatigue-related conditions.

Located in London's prestigious Harley Street, the Optimum Health Clinic (OHC) had established an outstanding reputation for innovation and excellence. I was also in demand as a public speaker and had been offered my own BBC TV series, which was, rather ironically, called *Panic Room*. On the surface I was leading a glamorous life, driving a sports car, and living in a penthouse apartment in London. And, given that I'd been mercilessly bullied throughout my school years, I was also proud to be dating the kind of women I could once only have dreamed of.

However, by the time I joined the retreat for a second time, I'd walked away from the TV series, given up my apartment, sold my car, and was living a hermit's existence, just trying to survive. If there was any chance that this retreat might help me, I had to stay with it. I could either continue living in a state of constant fear and anxiety or finally face up to my emotions. Both options felt impossible, but I knew I had to do *something*.

Emotional Shutdown

When I reached the far side of the forest, I slowed my pace a little, gazing at the mist lingering over the mountains in the distance. As I walked on, I found myself reflecting on my childhood and how some of the events that had occurred back then had shaped my current life. I realized that, ultimately, my inability to feel my emotions must have been a natural response to the traumas I'd experienced during my early years.

The word trauma didn't mean a great deal to me at that time. I thought of trauma as the physical injuries sustained in a serious accident or, say, the experience of living in a war zone. The idea that the childhood I'd normalized had been 'traumatic' seemed strange to me. I knew that many people had experienced far more difficult things than I had, and yet I did recognize that the shutting down of my emotional capacity must have originated somewhere.

From a young age, my sister suffered from significant mental health issues. Severe anorexia and bipolar disorder were the diagnoses at the time, but those labels did little to capture the lived experience for her and those around her. She spent periods in mental health hospitals and foster care, and although her own pain was intense, the effects of her illness on the family and others were also devastating.

I have countless childhood memories of my sister being violent toward family members and smashing up the house. And on multiple occasions I sat in the back of a police car with her, trying to soothe her as she was once again taken into enforced residential care.

Growing up with someone whose feelings were so explosive and destructive, I'd learned a clear lesson: Emotions are dangerous and the more we express them, the more we and those around us get hurt. The problem was that now, on the retreat, I was being asked to open up to and feel my feelings, but they were simply not accessible to me. And the closer I got to them, the more severe the panic and terror became. Never in my life had I felt more stuck.

Taking a Leap

Later that day, I had a private session with one of the retreat's teachers. These were designed to help us integrate the theory of the teaching into our everyday experience, but so far, I'd generally seen them as something to get through, and certainly not a place in which to be truly vulnerable.

My teacher, Prakash, was a stocky Glaswegian in his late fifties whose voice was a bit like Sean Connery's. When he wasn't teaching retreats, he lived in Hawaii, and I'd been having online video sessions with him for the past year. During that time, we'd talked a lot about my growing predicament of emotional 'stuckness,' but I'd not managed to move beyond it.

As I sat with Prakash and updated him on how the week had been for me, he listened patiently and empathically. When I was finished, he regarded me with a stern but compassionate look in his eyes and said, 'Alex, I think the time for talking is done.' He then invited me to lie on a mat on the floor and close my eyes. I did as I was told, even though a huge part of me once again wanted to pack my bags and run. But I feared that if I did, I might spend the rest of my life running, and that wouldn't be a life worth living.

Prakash asked me to put my focus on my breath and to pay attention to the sensations in my body; in doing so, he was encouraging me to deepen my focus on my inner experience and to give up trying to control it. At first, I felt nothing but the familiar stuckness and hopelessness. But then, as I felt into the feelings, to my surprise I noticed something else was there, and one word came to mind to describe it: *hatred*.

The feeling was mainly in my chest, but it was growing. It felt cold and toxic, and it was almost as if there was a demonic force rising within me. It occurred to me that I might be about to get more than I'd bargained for. Prakash suggested I stay with the feeling, and I realized that this was a pivotal moment. If I'd really decided that my life couldn't continue in the way it was, I had to dig deep and grow my courage. I allowed the feeling of hatred to spread more fully into my body, and as I did so, I started to get images of my father. I say images, but they were more vague ideas of what he might look like – I'd grown up without my father and had only ever seen two photographs of him.

As I did my best to continue to allow the feeling, it started to build. I knew that there would be a tipping point, when the control would no longer be mine, and I gave myself over to the feeling and to Prakash's guidance. As someone who was used to being in control, this wasn't easy for me. The tipping point arrived, and before I knew it, I'd taken a leap.

Suddenly, out of nowhere, the feeling of hatred became overwhelming. It was like a poison infecting every cell of my body. I began to scream, making the most murderous sounds I'd ever heard. And one phrase, on repeat, came out of my mouth between those screams, as if they were the only words I knew: 'I hate him. I hate him. I hate him so much.'

By then, my entire body was shaking intensely, and at one point, I thought I'd be sick. For a moment, I found myself wondering what the hell was happening. Where had all this intensity come from? Thankfully, my years of meditation practice had taught me to stay present in difficult circumstances, and I knew that if ever there was a time to keep my attention steady, this was it.

Our Pain Is the Gateway to Our Healing

Until I was in my early twenties, it had barely crossed my mind that my father leaving the family soon after I was born had impacted me in any way. It wasn't until I stumbled across a weekend workshop on exploring family dynamics that I was faced with the undeniable truth – my father walking out had been a defining event of my life.

I wasn't aware of the circumstances of my parents' separation, but I did know that my conception had been a failed attempt to save their marriage; indeed, they had even argued about what to call me. Eventually, my mother divorced my father on grounds of mental cruelty. He stopped visiting us a few months after the divorce was finalized, and we had no contact with him at all after I was about six months old.

My father didn't just leave us physically, he also left us financially, failing to pay a penny in child support. As a result, at one point my mother had to work three jobs to support my sister and me. At a young age, I became the man of the house – I had to be strong, and when my sister lost one of her ongoing battles with her mental health, I was often the person who tried to make it better. And, despite being one of the most bullied kids in my school, I'd still try to protect other kids from bullies by standing between them. I couldn't bear to see other people suffer – to see them feeling the pain that I felt, deep down.

Alongside the physical and emotional stress of the events of my childhood, I learned something deeply formative: the pain I was experiencing was my fault. As children we are egocentric – we believe the world revolves around us, and, more importantly, is *caused* by us. Therefore, the trauma that happens to us – be it a parent leaving, or other emotional instability we experience – must, on some level, be our own fault. Right?

As I lay on the floor in that retreat center, with Prakash kneeling over me and my body trying to purge itself of the poison that was consuming me, for the first time I understood the difference between anger and hatred. Anger has a fiery, hot quality, while hatred is cold. I didn't just want my father dead, I wanted to kill him, and I wanted it to be slow and cruel. I wanted to hurt him in every way that he'd hurt us.

I knew there was a good chance that my father was still alive. So why had he never reached out? At the very least, he could have checked to see if we were OK. There had been nothing – not a single phone call or letter. It *hurt*. It hurt so much.

After what felt like an eternity but was probably closer to 15 minutes, the hatred in me began to dissipate a little. Prakash gently asked me what I was feeling now. At first, I hesitated. I desperately didn't want it to be true, but I knew that my hatred was really a defense against something even more painful: I wanted my father. I needed him. More than anything in the world, I desperately longed for my father to love me.

In hating my father, I experienced the illusion of power, but in *feeling* my need for him, it was as if I had no defenses left. As Prakash softly encouraged me to continue to allow my feelings, the sensations in my heart were so intense, it felt as if it was breaking.

As my hatred turned to sadness, my screams dissolved into desperate sobs. As tears poured down my cheeks, I became the little boy whose father had abandoned him. The little boy who was utterly innocent, yet believed, on some level, that it was his fault. The little boy who needed the love of his father like he needed food and oxygen. It was a pain that nothing in the world could heal. The love of a father seemed, to me, to be the most basic human right, and I couldn't have it.

The Beauty of Surrender

I felt that I was in a place from which I could never return, and with a heartbreak so absolute and so final. But then, something totally unexpected happened. From the depths of my broken heart, a new feeling started to arise: love. My broken heart began to transform into the deepest and most all-consuming feeling of love I'd ever experienced.

I was beyond logic and rationality at this point, so I didn't even begin to try to make sense of it. I just followed Prakash as he used his words and loving presence to guide me deeper into what was happening. As this new feeling continued to build, I had no resistance left. It was as if my heart was the center of a vortex of pure, unconditional love. It wasn't love for someone or something; it was just love. It was as if love was the fabric of everything and everyone. My heart still ached, but not in a way that hurt; instead, it felt utterly exquisite, and the feeling vibrated through every cell of my being.

As Prakash encouraged me to breathe into the feeling more and more, my conscious mind almost entirely dropped away. It wasn't even that I was consumed by the love. I *was* the love. I *was* bliss. It was everything that we spend lifetimes searching for, there and then, in that moment, lying on the floor of a retreat center.

What I'd discovered at the heart of my deepest pain and trauma was the exact opposite of what I'd feared. My emotions were not something to fear and escape from; in learning to trust and open to them, I'd unleashed their innate wisdom for healing.

Real Change Takes Time

Now, if life was like a Hollywood movie, from that moment of inner breakthrough I'd have lived happily ever after. But in reality, things were rather bumpier. Having cracked open my heart, I spent much of the next six months feeling ragingly angry. From engaging in intense weight lifting sessions to screaming into numerous innocent pillows, it was an ongoing process to move the stored energy from my body.

Then, just as it seemed that the anger and hatred had cleared, I went through a further six months of sadness and despair. I'd burst into tears at my desk at work, in the middle of yoga classes, and many other inconvenient and embarrassing places.

But as my journey of healing my trauma unfolded, my life transformed with it. Almost immediately, my panic attacks stopped as my nervous system came back into balance. Eventually, my relationship with myself and my emotions changed. And a few years later, following a lengthy period of frustrating dating and an inability to stay with anyone for longer than a few months, I met Tania, the woman who would become my wife, and was able to have a very different kind of relationship – one built on emotional depth and connection.

In time, my working life also became deeply informed by my inner experiences; they were a key factor in the Therapeutic Coaching® model I created, which remains at the core of everything I do today. Therapeutic Coaching focuses on healing the impacts of our past traumas, creating the future we want, but ultimately learning to live in the now.

Our Work Together

Since you're reading this book, there's a good chance that you've experienced emotional trauma of some kind. Perhaps the traumas that have shaped you and your life are clear to you, or perhaps right now they aren't. It may be that your traumas are far more severe than my own, and it may be the opposite and you think you 'have nothing to complain about.'

However, as we'll soon discuss, *all* our experiences matter, and part of our work together in this book will be to decode your childhood experiences and understand how their impact has echoed through your life. In the coming chapters, my aim isn't only to help you understand how your past has shaped you and teach you how to heal it, but also to show you what's likely preventing you from doing so.

Indeed, often the challenge isn't what's caused us pain but what's in the way of healing it. As we'll explore, as a direct result of trauma, our body and nervous system go into the exact opposite of the state they need to be in to heal. Furthermore, this is often nuanced and tricky territory; for example, there's a huge difference between feeling your emotions and throwing them at other people. Ultimately, our goal is to create more love and connection in your life, not less.

And healing your trauma isn't only about some big breakthrough, like the one I've just described. Although such advances might happen along the way, what's far more important is your day-to-day emotional connection, how you relate to yourself, and the place from which you meet the world around you. If your relationship with yourself is difficult, you'll find that every other relationship in your life is affected, too.

So much of what we struggle with in life comes from a deep sense of inner shame and judgement. What sits at the heart of our healing is a pivotal shift in our relationship with ourselves. We must realise that whatever happened, or didn't happen, to us in childhood wasn't our fault. I wasn't to blame when my father left, or when my family felt like it was disintegrating around me. The events that shaped you are *not your fault*. The idea that we are responsible for these events is not only fundamentally incorrect, but is corrosive and extremely damaging.

An important step towards healing is to own our feelings towards our parents. We can recognise that our parents likely did care about and love us, but this isn't the same as having the skills and capacity to truly meet our developmental needs.

In this book, we are going to contextualise and make sense of how your childhood trauma has affected you, but our journey together doesn't end there. While we are utterly unable to change the events of our formative years, our *healing* from those events is ultimately our responsibility. If we want the circumstances of our lives as adults to change, we are responsible for changing them. True freedom in life comes from understanding what has shaped us, but also doing the work to break free.

Having worked with thousands of patients over the years, as well as leading one of the largest clinical teams in the world specializing in complex chronic illnesses, one thing is fundamentally true to me: healing on all levels is possible. It can take time, and it can be very hard work, but your efforts will bring you gifts beyond your imagination.

Using This Book

It's Not Your Fault is organized into three parts.

- In **Part I**, we'll decode your trauma and look at the ways that it echoes in your life.

- In **Part II**, you'll learn the RESET model for creating change in your nervous system.

- In **Part III**, we'll delve into the ABCD of trauma healing in the real world of our relationships with others and committing to lasting change.

I'm pleased to offer a free online companion course to help you dive deeper into healing your trauma. In this, you'll find interviews with many of the trauma experts who have inspired my ideas, filmed therapy sessions with some of the case studies I share, and practical tools to help bring the book to life. You can access the companion course at www.alexhoward.com/trauma.

I'd also like to say a few words about the tone I've used in the book. I hope that you'll feel supported and held by me through my choice of language. At times, I also hope to challenge you or help you to see things that you may feel some resistance to seeing. As I say to my patients, our work together should always feel safe, but it may not always feel comfortable. If this is the case for you, please remember that I challenge you with only the best of intentions.

Finally, I'd like to thank you for trusting me to be your guide. I don't take you investing your hope and your heart lightly, and equally, in my wish to meet you where you are on your journey, I've poured my heart into this book and living its tools in my own life.

As it quickly became clear to me while I was writing *It's Not Your Fault*, if I want to invite you to have an honest dialogue with yourself about your trauma, the most powerful way is to share some of the gifts I've received in doing that same process myself. And, like all of us, I am of course a work in progress! So, let's get started – let's explore what trauma really is, and how it echoes in our lives.

CHAPTER 2

Trauma as an ECHO

It was a beautiful evening in early summer, and I was taking a much-needed walk in the Hampshire Downs in Southeast England. A few months earlier, the COVID-19 pandemic had begun and, faced with being confined to our London home with three energetic young girls, my wife and I had made a dash for the countryside. We found a house for rent on Airbnb and arrived there with a van full of our possessions the following day.

In our new location, life was an odd seesaw, our blissful family time contrasting with the difficult challenges of home schooling two children with neurodivergent learning needs and entertaining a toddler who was desperate to play with other children.

My working life was an exciting but intense combination of seeing patients online, teaching our Therapeutic Coaching® practitioner training, overseeing my various businesses, and writing a book about my work with fatigue-related illnesses. I also found myself producing an online conference on trauma.

I'd already hosted an online event on fatigue for more than 40,000 participants, and with trauma being a key part of my clinical work, as well as an area that connects mind–body healing with functional medicine, it had seemed the obvious next step. And so, the Trauma Super Conference was born.

In preparation, I spent a few months recording interviews with many of the world's leading experts on trauma, including Dr. Gabor Maté, Dr. Peter Levine, and Professor Stephen Porges. The process was fascinating as I always enjoy the opportunity to dive deep into others' work and expand my own knowledge.

However, in more recent weeks, I'd also been experiencing a growing sense of shock, and that evening as I climbed higher in the hills, the sun setting in the sky, the enormity of what was happening around the world started to hit me.

A Peaking Wave

The inaugural Trauma Super Conference had attracted more than 185,000 attendees. In fact, so many people had tried to access it on the first day, our website had gone down for 10 hours. As I continued my walk, I began to question why it had been one of the biggest online conferences in internet history.

It could partly be explained by the enormous suffering caused by COVID-19 lockdowns, and by the huge numbers of people who'd been affected by and/or had lost loved ones to the virus, as well as the collective trauma of living through a pandemic; another factor was the dialogue on trauma and race inequality catalyzed by the murder of George Floyd.

But to me, it also felt as if a wave that had been building for many years had finally peaked and in my position at the helm of the Trauma Super Conference, I just happened to be at the heart of it. After the event, there were thousands of comments on Facebook and our email program crashed several times, responding as though the many legitimate emails we received each day were a spam attack.

That afternoon, I'd read just a few of those emails, and each one contained a story that moved me deeply. There was Rachel from Texas who'd lost her daughter in a car crash caused by a drink driver the previous year and was battling unimaginable grief that manifested as intense anxiety and depression. There was Tony in Melbourne who'd been sexually abused as a child and had only recently come to terms with the fact it was blocking intimacy with his wife some 30 years later. Then there was Kiara in Mumbai who'd been orphaned at birth and was trying to understand why she constantly felt the need to self-medicate her emotional pain.

The first Trauma Super Conference had been attended by people in 169 countries, and it revealed one overwhelming truth – trauma affects people in every nation, regardless of their sex, age, privilege, or background. And, as you'll soon see, trauma comes in many forms, and it can affect us in numerous different ways.

What Is Trauma?

In the simplest terms, trauma is an injury that doesn't heal. In this book, we'll primarily be talking about emotional trauma from early childhood, although the impacts of this trauma can be felt at any time in life. And, as we'll explore, what we learned in childhood is a key factor in determining how we respond to life's blows as an adult.

When the emotional injuries of our lives don't heal, the feelings and emotions that are triggered must go somewhere. One way of understanding this is to imagine that we're all walking around with a big black sack stuffed with unprocessed and undigested life experiences. Sometimes the sack is sealed tight, while at other times its top comes off with predictable frequency.

Here's a classic example of the latter. We're driving along a road in a seemingly neutral and relaxed frame of mind, lost in our thoughts and half listening to a podcast, when another driver cuts us off on the inside, forcing us to brake suddenly to avoid hitting them. In that moment, we have an explosion of anger, and must restrain ourselves from catching up with the driver and instigating a fight to the death.

What just happened? How did we go from chilled pussycat to full-blown Conor McGregor in the space of a few moments? Well, it's likely that an unprocessed emotional injury inside us just got rubbed with some salt. Perhaps, during our childhood, we experienced the trauma of not being seen, or of always being told that we didn't deserve to take our place. Whatever it was, the proverbial top on that black sack of emotions was lifted, and the unprocessed trauma exploded out.

Now, you might be thinking to yourself, *Yes Alex, that's all well and good, but that lunatic did just cut me off.* To which I'd respond, it's true that they were driving badly, but perhaps they had a good reason to do so, such as rushing to help a loved one in distress. But the point here isn't *their* behavior, but why something so explosive just happened in *you*.

So, trauma is unprocessed emotion in our body caused by an unprocessed emotional experience... and it's also a little more complex than that. For some people this unhealed, unprocessed injury is an obvious one – for example, they once experienced a traumatic event such as being physically attacked and having to fight, and now whenever they're out alone their nervous system goes into panic. For others it might be a more subtle event, such as being laughed at in the classroom for saying the wrong thing, which resulted in a fear of public speaking.

The Importance of Emotional Resilience

However, by itself, the emotional event isn't enough to determine whether we experience trauma. Indeed, using the previous example, for some people fighting is their greatest thrill and they dedicate their lives to mastering the mixed martial arts or boxing; and there are those who have found great joy in being able to make others laugh.

So, although trauma requires a trigger *event*, that alone isn't enough to determine whether trauma happens. The *context* within which the event takes place is also critical. How those around us, and we ourselves, respond to the event has a huge impact.

We have three core emotional needs – boundaries, safety, and love. If these emotional needs are met by our caregivers during our early development, and in time, we're taught how to meet them for ourselves, they help us to develop a kind of resilience that will significantly reduce our likelihood of being traumatized as we journey through life.

For example, if we're taught how to have (and are allowed) healthy boundaries, we develop an 'emotional immune system' that protects us from the world around us. If we're taught how to self-regulate our nervous system to feel safe, we're able to process the shocks that happen to us in life. And a deep sense of love and feeling lovable acts like a healing antidote to the events which might hit us.

Conversely, if our three core emotional needs are not met by our caregivers and we don't therefore have the emotional resilience they provide, when we find ourselves experiencing potentially traumatic events, over time, it leads to a *shift* in the *homeostatic balances* in our body. The impact of these homeostatic shifts on our physical and emotional well-being is enormous. By living on edge in anticipation of future trauma events which may never occur, we create our own vicious cycle of suffering.

These *outcomes* of our trauma can themselves further perpetuate the cycle of suffering. Perhaps we learn that to be lovable, we need to be the best at everything we do, or maybe our sense of self-worth comes from constantly giving to and being there for others, even to our detriment.

As I explained in the last chapter when I talked about my journey, often, the true suffering of the trauma is not the events themselves but the shifts in our nervous system and the outcomes in terms of the way we respond and live. After all, my long run of disastrous relationships wasn't caused by the actual events of my childhood, but by the coping strategies I'd created to try to escape them.

ECHO: The Four Stages of Trauma

As you can see, trauma is so much more than just an event. Trauma is a series of stages that we go through. In my own reflections, one helpful discovery I made is that there are in fact four stages of trauma, and we've just touched on them:

1. The Event

2. The Context

3. The Homeostatic shift

4. The Outcomes in our lives

To help unpack this ECHO way of thinking about trauma, let's look briefly at these stages through the lens of my trauma.

1: The Event

Traumatic events can be single or repetitive events; they can be routine experiences; and they can be one-off moments. For some people the traumas of their life are obvious, while for others they're much less so. Ultimately, though, for trauma to happen, there must be a trigger event that in some way creates an overload in the nervous system.

In my case, there were two major trigger events. The first was being abandoned as a baby by my father, and the second was a series of experiences with my sister and her severe mental health issues. These were intense and overwhelming experiences that presented a significant challenge for my emotional body to process (we'll talk about the emotional body soon.)

2: The Context

Two people can experience the same event, but one is traumatized by it and the other isn't. This is because two people can experience the same event and respond to it completely differently due to the internal and external context within which it happens. How we, and the people around us, respond to an event ultimately determines whether there's trauma or not.

The way that we respond to an event is determined by our emotional resilience and our capacity to work through and process the shocks of life. And our emotional resilience is driven by whether our three core emotional needs were met early in our life (we'll talk more about emotional resilience in Chapter 4.)

As children we're dependent on those around us to meet these emotional needs for us; and as adults we can learn to meet them for ourselves. A key factor in determining how well we learn to meet our needs is how well they were (or weren't) met for us as children.

We'll dive into this in more detail later, but here's a brief overview of our three core emotional needs:

- Boundaries: Our boundaries with others give us the ability to say no and protect ourselves. Our boundaries with ourselves define our ability to self-discipline and motivate ourselves to follow through.

- Safety: Our physical and emotional safety and our capacity to self-regulate our nervous system will determine whether trauma is held in our body.

- Love: This is the oxygen that sustains our emotional body. When we have an emotional injury, love is the antidote that helps us to heal.

In my case, with my father leaving and my mother's boundaries being heavily violated by the nature of their divorce, there was no caregiver able to hold boundaries for me. The trauma in my mother's nervous system – a result of all that was going on in her life – meant that her ability to co-regulate and to soothe me was impaired. And although I knew I was loved by my mother, my father didn't love me enough to hang around.

And in terms of the trauma of my sister's mental health issues, her behavior was so extreme it smashed any boundaries and created a constant sense that there were no safe places; the nervous systems of everyone around me were constantly on edge, and again, although there was love, it was polluted by the chaos that surrounded me.

3: The Homeostatic Shift

Trauma causes changes in our body. When our nervous system becomes overloaded, our body's stress response, which is designed to keep us safe when we're under immediate threat, becomes stuck in the 'on' mode. I call this a maladaptive stress response and we pay a heavy price in our physical and emotional well-being in maintaining this mode.

Over time, a maladaptive stress response leads to shifts in the various homeostatic balances in our body (we'll talk about this in detail in Chapter 5.) This means that a state of anxiety, which might at one time in our evolution have been necessary for our survival, becomes our normalized way of being.

In my case, the overwhelm caused by my father leaving and the subsequent chain of events, along with my sister's constant emotional outbursts, meant that my nervous system was conditioned toward living in a maladaptive stress response. The crippling anxiety I experienced later in my life, which I described earlier, was a big part of this. However, the constant stress overload was also my body's attempt to escape my feelings, which I was terrified of experiencing.

4: The Outcomes in Our Lives

Having experienced the events of trauma, along with the resulting homeostatic shifts in our nervous system due to our core emotional needs of boundaries, safety, and love not being met, there are, inevitably, outcomes. Our life becomes heavily influenced by our attempts to find ways to meet our three core emotional needs – not only to heal our past but also to unlock our future and live more easily in the present.

For example, if we learned that the only way to get our emotional need of love met is by constantly achieving and being the best at everything we do, that will become our modus operandi. Or perhaps we learned that the best way to feel safe is to continually try to control ourselves and the world around us.

My experience was that my sense of self-worth and my ability to meet my core emotional needs of safety and love were tied not only to what I achieved but also to being the rescuer and helper for other people. Constantly being there for others was more important than being there for myself, and my feelings were my greatest fear.

We're Wired to Heal

What I believe is so important about the ECHO way of thinking about our trauma is that it clearly highlights that our real suffering isn't the event or events that have already happened in the past, but what happens in our nervous system in response, and the outcomes in our lives as we manage this. Indeed, although the origin of our trauma may lie decades earlier, the ECHOs are very much reverberating now.

The good news is that this is a huge message of hope. After all, we can't change what happened in the past, but we can certainly transform how it's impacting our experiences and choices in life now. And that's the work we'll do together in this book.

Now, as vital as it is that you understand your personal journey with trauma and how you've responded to it, what really matters is how we unlock your capacity to heal. Indeed, at the heart of this book is the premise that our emotional body has a natural capacity to heal; in fact, it's wired to do so.

Our Emotional Body

Along with our physical body, we have an emotional body, which is home to our emotions and feelings. When we feel angry or sad, joyful or excited, the seat of these emotions is our emotional body.

If you get a wound in your physical body, provided you keep it clean (and if necessary, have your skin stitched together), your body will heal it. The same is true if you break a bone – as long as you avoid aggravating it, the bone will heal itself. Your doctor might prescribe painkillers to help you manage the pain, and they might put the bone in a cast to keep it still, but the healing comes from within the miracle of your being.

The same is true of emotional wounds, or trauma. Our emotional body has a natural capacity for healing, provided we create the conditions for the healing mechanism to do its work. To put it bluntly: Whatever you've experienced, however horrific it might have been at the time, and despite the ECHOs in your life feeling like a deafening wall of sound that you can't ignore, even for a second, *healing is possible.* You. Can. Heal.

However, for the natural capacity of our emotional healing to kick in, certain conditions must be met. In a sense you need to learn to become the loving, skillful, and well-resourced caregiver you perhaps never had. It might take time, and it most likely won't be a straight line, but you can do it.

So, now that we've taken a brief walk through the four stages, or ECHOs, of trauma let's take a closer look at the first stage: the *events* of your trauma.

CHAPTER 3

Discover Your Trauma Events

We've all had a first true love in life – a person or a thing that we became obsessed with and found ourselves thinking about every spare minute of every day. For me, it was psychology. And, like many obsessive love affairs, my love of psychology was born out of pain, desperation, and the belief that I'd finally found the antidote to my misery.

After two years of suffering from a severe chronic illness that had devastated my life to the point where I seriously questioned whether I wanted to continue living it, I stumbled across a book called *Way of the Peaceful Warrior* by Dan Millman, and soon after that, Louise Hay's classic *You Can Heal Your Life*.

I say stumbled, but in truth, my grandmother had left these books in a strategic place, hoping I might pick them up. She was wise enough to realize that given my stubborn nature if she told me to read them there was little chance I would. But pain plus hope is a powerful combination, and for me, it equaled change.

These two books gave me hope that there might be a different way to live, and they also opened my eyes to a whole new universe of what my life might mean and the choices I had to potentially change it. In the ensuing months I read more intensely and widely, quickly exhausting the self-help books my grandmother owned. Eventually, I had to make a rather embarrassing trip to the local library to borrow more (as an 18-year-old male asking for books on self-love, I got some strange looks.)

A year later, my health had recovered sufficiently for me to go to university, and there was only one thing I wanted to study: psychology. A few weeks into my course, however, I discovered that the mainstream psychology approach wasn't going to meet my desire to find more innovative and experimental ways of working. And so, hungry for more, in my spare time I continued to read self-help books, along with attending additional workshops and courses whenever possible.

Adverse Childhood Experiences (ACEs)

Walking this path alone for the first few years was lonely and difficult, and I was deeply grateful for the friendships and connections that began to emerge. Simply having people to talk to and share new discoveries and reflections with was like nectar for my soul.

One particular friend at the time, Katie, was on her own chronic illness healing journey; she'd walked away from a successful career in media to retrain and pursue her dream of becoming a psychologist. Together, we tried to make sense of our current physical and emotional challenges, and during one of our many conversations we talked about the impact of our past.

Had our childhood played a role in our current health difficulties? Put another way, what had been the effects of Adverse Childhood Experiences – potentially traumatic events that occur in childhood?

In the mid-1980s a groundbreaking study[1] was carried out by Kaiser Permanente, a US-based insurance company that provides its services for a fixed fee and is therefore highly motivated to maintain and protect the health of its members to reduce its long-term liability. One of the key programs offered by Kaiser Permanente at the time was an obesity treatment program, and the company had observed that although most participants successfully lost weight while following this, the dropout rate was 50 percent.

The head of the company's preventative medicine department, Vincent Felitti, became intensely curious about the reasons for this and decided to interview a selection of the participants who had quit the program. What he discovered would shape the world of trauma research for decades to come.

Of the 286 people Felitti spoke to, the vast majority had been sexually abused as children. This led him to wonder whether their weight gain might in fact be a coping mechanism for the depression, anxiety, and fear they reported experiencing. He teamed up with Robert Anda from the US's Centers for Disease Control and Prevention (CDC), and together they studied the childhood trauma experiences of more than 17,000 volunteers.

The Three Types of ACEs

Along the way, Felitti and Anda coined the term Adverse Childhood Experiences, or ACEs, which they defined as 'potentially traumatic events that can have negative, lasting effects on health and well-being.' They determined that ACEs fall into three categories – abuse, neglect, and household dysfunction; here's an overview of what these are:

Abuse
- Physical abuse
- Emotional abuse
- Sexual abuse

Neglect
- Physical neglect
- Emotional neglect

Household Dysfunction

- Mental illness in the household
- Mother treated violently
- Divorce of parents
- Incarcerated relative
- Substance abuse in the family

The study discovered that ACEs are common – 28 percent of the study participants reported physical abuse and 21 percent sexual abuse – and they also occur together: Almost 40 percent of those interviewed reported two or more ACEs, and 12.5 percent reported four or more.

In the decades since this important study, a substantial body of follow-up research has served to further confirm these findings.[2–5] What's perhaps most shocking is that those who have six or more ACEs have on average a 20-year reduction in their life span.

Covert Trauma

As my friend Katie and I reflected on our childhoods, for me, the events of my trauma were fairly obvious – my early years' experiences formed an almost perfect list of ACEs. My parents had divorced; I'd been abandoned by my father; my sister had suffered from serious mental illness and was violent; alcohol was used as a coping strategy in the family; and at times we'd experienced considerable financial hardship.

Katie, on the other hand, had experienced a seemingly more positive childhood. Her parents were still married, and she had a good relationship with her sister and her wider family. Her parents both worked hard and contributed financially to the household, which meant that although money wasn't abundant, there was enough. Katie had been popular at school, had good friends, and later developed a successful career.

That was until, like me, she was forced onto a complex and challenging healing journey.

With a childhood which on the surface was a happy one, how could Katie claim to have been emotionally wounded? Indeed, she said it felt self-indulgent and disrespectful to people with 'real' trauma to even consider that her 'happy childhood' had affected her negatively. And yet, she had many of the same struggles that I did. Beyond living with a chronic illness, she also suffered with anxiety and low mood at times, and for several years had felt that her life lacked purpose and meaning. Like so many of us, Katie believed that she was broken and, on some level, that it was her fault.

Digging a little beneath the surface, the origins of Katie's pain began to reveal themselves. Although her parents loved her, they were themselves not emotionally open. And as an emotional and sensitive child, Katie hadn't known what to do with her feelings. She was taught they were a sign of weakness that had to be overcome; indeed, she'd regularly say things like, 'Ignore me, I'm just being overly emotional.'

The more we explored together, the more we realized that in fact Katie's childhood had impacted her as intensely as mine had – it was just that those impacts were more subtle and hidden. In a sense, the fact that she hadn't explicitly experienced ACEs in the way I had, made them even more difficult to identify and work with.

Forms of Covert Trauma

Many years later I came to label experiences such as divorce, being abandoned, living with family members with mental illness and so on as *overt trauma* – i.e., they're obviously traumatic experiences. The more subtle and insidious experiences, such as those that Katie had experienced, I'd refer to as *covert trauma* – they're not necessarily less harmful in their impact, but they're often harder to see.[6] Although there are many different forms of covert trauma, here are a few examples:

- Not feeling emotionally seen or validated in your own emotions. This might be being told, like Katie, that 'You're just being emotional – get over it.'

- Being taught that your self-worth is tied to what you do/achieve. Maybe you weren't top of the class in a subject at school and were told this meant you'd failed and were stupid.

- Not feeling attuned to, recognized by, seen, or validated by your caregivers, or not connecting with peers, because your experience of the world is so different to theirs and they don't understand you. For example, you may be neurodivergent and your lived experience is different to theirs.

- Learning that other people's needs are more important than your own. For example, routinely being told to ignore what you want and prioritizing those around you.

- Being made to feel ashamed of your race or heritage. For example, being part of a minority ethnic group in your hometown and being bullied for it by other children.

- Not receiving the same amount of love/attention from your parents as your siblings.

- Your parents being physically or emotionally absent due to other priorities, such as work or hobbies, which made you feel that everything else was more important than you.

Obviously, this is far from an exhaustive list, and we'll dig more into covert trauma as we continue our journey.

One-Time Versus Recurrent Traumatic Events

I think it's also helpful to make a distinction between events that happened once and those that became almost routine in our childhood. Although a single event can be a major source of trauma, when something becomes a repetitive experience, it has the additional cost of becoming normalized.

For example, as a child, seeing our parents have a heated argument once can be upsetting, but if our core emotional needs are being met appropriately, it might be a helpful insight into the realities of managing conflict and differences of opinion. But if witnessing our parents argue becomes the norm, the impact is very different. Our nervous system will learn to activate to help us brace ourselves for the shocks, and we'll normalize to this new homeostatic balance.

Is It Normal Not to Remember Traumatic Events?

As you're reading this, you might be starting to think of the various events of your childhood that you believe have impacted you. If so, that's great, as you're one step ahead already. However, it's also entirely possible that you're feeling lost because you have a patchy recollection of your childhood at best.

If this is the case, you're most definitely not alone. Indeed, multiple research studies have demonstrated the impact of early trauma on our memories of childhood.[7-11] As we'll get into in Chapter 6, one of the ways we manage the impacts of our trauma is by learning to avoid and distract ourselves from our emotions. At the stronger end of this response, we can have difficulty forming accurate memories at the time of the event.

Furthermore, there's also evidence of a link between trauma and a tendency to overgeneralize autobiographical memories rather than remember individual events.[12-17] For example, on being asked specifically to describe one occasion when we felt joy, we might say that we used to enjoy going to the fair, rather than talk about one occasion when we went to the fair.

In his important book *Trauma and Memory*[18] Dr. Peter Levine explores how the body can store traumatic memories as feelings and sensations rather than thoughts and ideas, and how we can use this understanding to process trauma in a different way, through what he calls Somatic (relating to the body) Experiencing.

What then often happens, during a safe and holding therapeutic process, is that those memories start to resurface.[19] This is a sign that the therapy is working, because our system now feels safe enough to offer the memories up for healing. That said, there's an ongoing debate in psychological circles about repressed and recovered memories and the accuracy of memories of historical traumatic events.[20-22] Therefore, I think it's important that we hold such memories carefully.

However, although the details of traumatic events in particular can be unreliable, the more central the information, the more likely it is that there are important elements of truth.[23,24] Therefore, if we do start to uncover memories of events for which we have no reference point in terms of whether or not they're true, we can work with the trauma and stored emotion, with a light holding of the details of all the facts.[25] At least until we can hopefully find some kind of external confirmation of them.[26]

In my work, I take the view that it's less about whether something is true, or objectively correct, but whether it feels real, and therefore there's some corresponding emotional trauma to be metabolized and processed, regardless. Indeed, my experience, both personally and professionally, is also that trauma can go into our body in one way and the memories that arise can be different from reality.

The Impact of Cultural Norms

Another consideration when trying to understand the life events that have shaped us is the cultural norms in the environment within which they happened. For example, let's say you grew up in a culture in which intellect was valued over emotional sensitivity, and expressing emotional needs was frowned upon. Perhaps this wasn't only the case in your home, but also in the church you attended, in your classroom at school, and at the heart of the way your society selected and celebrated the cultural icons it did. As a result, you came to believe that thoughts matter more than feelings.

However, just because this belief was normalized and shared by everyone around you, it doesn't reduce the impact of the event. In fact, it often worsens it because there was no support for the challenge that may well have instinctively been rising inside you to say you had a core emotional need that wasn't being met.

For people who are neurodivergent, such as those with autism or sensory, information, or attention issues such as ADHD or dyslexia, the experience of being misunderstood is all too common. The same is true for those whose sexual orientation hasn't been embraced, or whose gender identification has been rejected or judged by those around them. When our true identity and lived experience are the trigger for our core emotional needs of boundaries, safety, and love being withdrawn or violated, it can be deeply traumatic.

As the father of two neurodiverse children and the husband of a neurodiverse wife, I feel deeply passionate about the importance of recognizing and validating the differences between us. Not as things to 'learn to accept and live with,' but as qualities to celebrate for the gifts they can be. Indeed, the number of great artists, thinkers, and entrepreneurs in our history who were not neurotypical is staggering. And, unfortunately, many who grow up today in ways that don't fit the mold of the society around them have experienced significant traumas as a result.

There's also fascinating evidence emerging around how trauma is passed between generations.[27-32] Experiences that have happened to our ancestors live in our DNA, and are also passed on through the behaviors and norms of our environment, families, and communities.[33,34] My friend Thomas Hübl has written particularly elegantly about this in his book *Healing Collective Trauma.*[35]

Part of the difficulty of unraveling the impact of the events of our childhood and beyond, and the way they've shaped the meanings we've created in response to them, is getting a clear sense not of what we've normalized but what's 'healthy.' And to do this effectively we often have to take a step away from the blame game, as it can simply perpetuate the cycle of our own suffering.

We'll explore this further in Part II, but for now it's important to understand that we can recognize the key caregivers in our childhood as having failed to meet our core emotional needs, or indeed as being the unintentional instigators of events that wounded us, while still loving them and knowing that in their heart, they loved us.

This isn't about making certain behaviors, or the lack of, acceptable or right. Or about removing our right to stand up for causes that we're passionate about. Indeed, skillful activism to drive change in the world is what's behind so many of our leaps forward. And one of the great emotional stretches that emotional healing as an adult involves is the ability to simultaneously feel the rage and hatred in the little child in us for not getting what it needed, while the adult in us recognizes the love that may also have been there.

Put another way, we can acknowledge that it's not our fault, but it's also not our parents' fault. They may have acted in ways which wounded us, but it's unlikely this was intentional. Indeed, their inability to skilfully meet our emotional needs was likely the product of their own parents' inability to do so for them, and so on. The potential gift of our healing is to help break the cycle of trauma.

Does Trauma Occur Only in Childhood?

At this point you'd be forgiven for thinking that only events that happen in childhood are important, as that's where our attention's been focused. The reason I've done so is that childhood events are particularly impactful for a few reasons. Firstly, it's during the first seven years of our life that our personality is shaped and formed. Secondly, as a child we're utterly dependent on those around us to meet our emotional needs, but as an adult we do at least have the self-reflective capacity to meet our own emotions.

However, trauma can happen at any point in our lives, even if the way we respond to it has likely been set up in childhood and will stay that way until we actively work to change it. The bottom line is that if we carry an unprocessed emotional injury from an event, or series of events, that's happened to us, then there's trauma.

The event could be overt or covert, a single event, or a series of events; our memory of it may be accurate or not; it may have happened in a culture that normalized it or not; and it could happen at any age. Ultimately, what matters is the impact of the event on us, and whether that impact left a wound that hasn't yet healed.

What Have Been the Key Trauma Events in Your Life?

So, we've arrived at your first exercise. It would be easy at this point to keep reading and say to yourself, *I'll do that later*, but the danger is that you won't. For this book to be more than just an intellectual process, completing the exercises is critical. Put simply, knowledge is nice, but action creates change.

Do your best to answer the following questions. Consider this a short checklist of possible traumatic events; it's far from comprehensive, and if something comes to mind that isn't listed here, please add it. You'll find an easy-to-complete worksheet for this exercise, and all the others in this book, in your free online companion course at www.alexhoward.com/trauma.

ACEs/Overt Trauma

Abuse
- Have you experienced physical abuse?
- Have you experienced emotional abuse?
- Have you experienced sexual abuse?

Neglect
- Are you aware of having been physically neglected as a child?
- Are you aware of having been emotionally neglected as a child?

Household dysfunction
- Was there mental illness in the household you grew up in?
- Were either of your parents treated violently?
- Did your parents divorce or separate?
- Were any of your relatives imprisoned?
- Was there substance abuse in your family?

Covert Trauma

- As a child, did you feel emotionally seen and validated?
- Were you taught that your self-worth was tied to what you did, rather than being intrinsic to your value as a human being?
- Did you feel rejected for being different to others?
- Did you learn that other people's needs were more important than your own?
- Did you feel shamed by or judged for your heritage or background?

- Did you feel that you had an equal amount of love/attention from your parents as your siblings?

- Were your parents physically or emotionally absent due to their other commitments – for example, work or hobbies?

Go Gently

I'm curious about what you discovered from doing this exercise. You might be feeling clarity and relief through having started to make some sense of your life events. Equally, you might be feeling overwhelmed and shocked at the number of traumas that register for you.

Here's the important thing, though: Whatever you're feeling is OK. If you're judging or rejecting yourself for what you're feeling right now, it's that very response which is perpetuating your trauma cycle. Being gentle with yourself along the healing journey is in itself a sign of healing. Remember, it's not your fault.

Now that we've begun to explore some of the key traumatic events of your life, it's time to turn our attention to how you responded to them. We're going to dive into the three core emotional needs that are critical for developing emotional resilience.

CHAPTER 4

Context Is Everything

As a child I loved superhero movies and stories. The idea of someone possessing special powers that made their life easier to navigate and gave them the ability to do superhuman things was more than just intriguing, it spoke to something I felt I lacked: the ability to be resilient in the face of life's blows.

However, what I loved even more than superhero stories were the tales of seemingly normal people who developed extraordinary abilities through discipline and hard work. Superman may have been born with the ability to fly, but more incredible was someone like Iron Man, who built a super-powerful suit, or the Karate Kid, who through great mentorship acquired the ability to stand up to his tormentors. Put another way, I loved the idea that superpowers could be learned.

As someone who grew up being heavily knocked by life, and feeling deeply shaped by those impacts, for many years I searched for ways to heal my traumas and help make my life easier and more functional. I didn't realize it at the time, but a byproduct of my healing journey was that my emotional black sack became a lot emptier, making me less easily triggered (although I'm human, and it still happens!) And I also developed greater emotional resilience.

Today, I notice that many of the things I once found hard, I no longer do, and when life throws its challenges at me, I'm more easily able to navigate through them. And I don't mean in an emotionally detached or shut-down way, but by staying emotionally open and present and moving through the feelings with as little resistance as possible.

Our Three Core Emotional Needs

The point about resilience isn't that it necessarily means we experience fewer knocks in life, but that we're better able to handle them when they do happen. We develop the flexibility to be tough when we need to be tough, and equally to be gentle when we need to be gentle. Life's knocks move through us rather than getting stuck and held in our nervous system.

Ultimately, it's this emotional resilience that determines whether our homeostatic balance shifts and we develop destructive, long-term coping strategies to attempt to manage this shift. And I've come to realize that just as there are critical ingredients for feeding our physical body – such as food, oxygen, and sleep – there are critical ingredients for the healthy development of our emotional body. It's these ingredients that help fuel us to develop our emotional resilience.

As we discussed in Chapter 2, there are three core ingredients to emotional resilience which, as children, we're entirely dependent on our parents or other caregivers to provide for us, but as we grow older, in healthy development, we can learn to meet for ourselves. The reality is that when our three core emotional needs are not met, we don't learn how to be with our own emotions in a healthy way. When we're unable to process our emotions, we end up with trauma.

So, let's look in detail at these three core emotional needs that a child must receive to develop in a healthy way and go on to reach its potential. They are the need for boundaries, the need for safety, and the need to feel love.

And please note that these are *needs* not *wants*. These are not preferences in life to support our healthy functioning, they're essential for our basic development. They're as important to our emotional body as food and sleep are to our physical body.

The Need for Boundaries

A boundary is a real or imagined line that indicates the limit or extent of something. A boundary separates self and other, inside and outside, and one nation from another. Healthy boundaries are critical to the functioning of almost every system on planet Earth.

One simple example is the immune system of our physical body, where it's the job of our T cells to determine what's a native cell and what's a foreign invader. If the foreign cell is in any way a threat, our natural killer (NK) cells (which are from the same family as T cells) will respond quickly to protect us. Indeed, part of the way vaccinations work is in teaching our immune system how to better mount a protective response to a disease that crosses our boundary.

Just like our physical body, our emotional body also needs boundaries. It needs us to be able to say yes or no to people, experiences, or events. On the most fundamental level, as children these are boundaries to protect us from people or experiences that might harm us. However, early in our development as a child, we need to learn to take on this function for ourselves, as our own wishes and desires become clearer to us, and only we can know what they are.

In our development, we go through a few cycles where this is a psychological priority, the first of which is commonly referred to as 'the terrible twos.' This is when children are developing and practicing their 'no,' and it can often be at the expense of getting what they really want, because the experience of having their 'no' in the moment is developmentally more important.

Although it's a source of deep frustration to parents everywhere, children don't do what we *say*, they do what we *do*, as we're their model for how to move through the world. So, as parents it's almost impossible to teach children boundaries in any way other than modelling them for them.

And clear and predictable boundaries are a crucial ingredient for our feeling safe as a child. Furthermore, a parent who's willing to establish and hold a boundary, particularly when it's inconvenient to them, is ultimately sending the message, *I love you enough to hold this boundary.*

Of course, part of the great adventure of parenting is that the moments we need to be the most skillful and empathic are often those when we feel the least resourceful and the most like screaming ourselves. Indeed, children almost have a sixth sense for sniffing out vulnerability in their parents and exploiting it. So, what I'm about to say is in no way intended as blame; it's just a statement of how things are. Parents, please be gentle with yourself as you read this – and I'll do the same!

Establishing and Maintaining Healthy Boundaries

Children need strong, predictable, and consistent boundaries, held in a loving and sensitive way. Healthy boundaries teach us how to say yes and no to others, but also how to do the same for ourselves. If you've ever struggled with self-discipline – which in essence, is the ability to say yes or no to yourself – then the chances are you have an inner boundary issue.

As much as healthy boundaries need to be predictable and consistent, they also need to be responsive. When a boundary is constantly rigid and not sensitive to what it's holding, it feels cold and cruel. When a boundary is held firmly but with a little give and take, and acts in a way that feels loving and sensitive, we feel truly supported.

For example, we may create a boundary with a child that says they need to go to bed at a certain time, and we hold this boundary predictably and firmly. But let's say they've invited a friend for a sleepover and are having a riot together, their hearts bursting with joy. Shutting down the fun in a cold and insensitive way by holding the bedtime boundary is likely to unleash a world of rage. Equally, letting a child play until they can't stand straight will cause everyone pain the following day.

So, the boundary needs to be sensitive, proportionate, and lovingly implemented, which doesn't preclude an appropriately escalating enforcement if it isn't heeded. Ultimately, the boundary giver needs to be attuned to the child's emotional response, and to adapt and adjust the boundaries in a way that feels supportive and not crushing.

Boundaries are also like a muscle, and they grow by being exercised and challenged beyond their current comfort zone. This means that children need to have something to push against or challenge (such as being told 'no'), because it helps them to grow their own sense of strength and to develop their will. Once again, this challenge needs to be appropriate, considered, and responsive to how it lands with the child.

On the flip side, a child being told they can do something (which they want to do), that they have what it takes and should go for it, is also important because it gives them the strength not to just grow and expand in their life, but also to meet the challenges they'll inevitably face. In essence, there's a power to both no and yes being used in the right way.

Of course, if we put too much strain on a muscle, we'll injure ourselves, and the same is true of children. But growing courage and emotional strength does require appropriate challenge and the shaping of our sense of inner strength and capacity, which is why I believe the current trend of overly protecting children's comfort is doing more harm than good.

Ultimately, when we learn how to establish and maintain healthy boundaries, we're able to protect ourselves from potentially harmful situations, and when we do find ourselves in them, we'll find it easier to extract ourselves. And when it's time to commit to our own healing, we'll have the self-discipline to say no to the distractions that arise and yes to the new habits and behaviors that will most support us.

The Need for Safety

The human body's nervous system has two branches. The first is our sympathetic nervous system, which is designed to stimulate and activate our body for action. The second is our parasympathetic nervous system, whose job it is to rest, digest, and regenerate. When one system is activated, the other is deactivated. Both branches are necessary for survival, and a healthy balance between the two is at the heart of a healthy life, because too much of either has associated problems.

When we perceive danger in our inner or outer environment, our sympathetic nervous system is activated so we can fight or flight in response to it (we'll look at this further in the next chapter.) However, when this sense of danger is constant or consistently overwhelming, this healthy survival mechanism, or 'stress response,' becomes maladaptive, and our nervous system can become stuck in a prolonged state of over-activation.

Our inner sense of safety as children has both a physical and an emotional component. We need to feel safe in the actual physical environment we're in, but that alone isn't enough. We can know that we're not in physical danger yet feel emotionally unsafe. For example, if we're around someone who constantly makes us feel judged or criticized, or we have a parent who's emotionally unpredictable, our nervous system will become activated to protect us.

Sometimes the threat in the environment is real, and other times it's a perceived threat, but the impact on our nervous system is the same. Indeed, our brain doesn't distinguish between something that's real and something that's vividly imagined. Furthermore, as small children, we consider much of the world a threat, and rightly so: Everything from the family cat to the fireplace is a danger until we learn how to be safe around it.

What helps to soothe us in the face of these constant dangers is the comfort and holding from our primary caregivers. In the case of healthy development, when we feel scared, or the world feels overwhelming, we'll return to our caregivers so they can reassure and comfort us. The comfort of our caregivers isn't only in the physical protection of their embrace, there's also a regulation that happens between our nervous system and theirs.[1-4]

However, if the caregiver we return to is themself not in a calm and soothing state, rather than merging with the comfort we need we actually merge with more stress.[5-8] Furthermore, if they dismiss or chastise us for seeking that comfort and holding, we'll learn that the world isn't a safe place and that we're wrong for seeking safety, and as a result, we may 'shut down' emotionally.[9]

If our emotional need for safety isn't met when we're young, we'll find that as we get older, our nervous system's resilience is diminished because it isn't sufficiently conditioned to deal with life's blows.

The Need for Love

Just as plants need sunlight to give them life, human beings need love. There's a huge body of research which demonstrates that when children are not given enough love, it impacts their development in almost every way.[10-13]

And it's not just any kind of love that we need as children. It's a specific kind – the love that ultimately helps us develop emotional resilience is unconditional love. When we're raised to believe that our self-worth and value are linked to what we do and how we act, we end up on a dangerous treadmill of constantly chasing love, as opposed to relaxing into the knowing that it's there as a foundation at the heart of who we are.

As children, to truly feel loved, we need to feel that we're adored and loved in the deepest sense of the word. There are different ways of demonstrating and expressing love, but as always, the actions of caregivers are more powerful than their words.

One of the most powerful demonstrations of love is attention and interest. When a child knows that their caregiver is genuinely interested in them, that they want to and enjoy spending time with them, they will feel loved. And children are emotionally attuned – they can feel when a parent is going through the motions but not truly giving them their interest and attention.

Furthermore, words and actions alone are not enough. As children we also need to *feel* love, which means responsive and affectionate human touch that respects our boundaries when we express them. If we're not touched and held as a child, and in age-appropriate ways as we mature, all the words and actions in the world may not be enough for us to truly feel that we're loved.[14–19]

Feeling a sense of physical and emotional love is also not enough. As a child we need to feel special. We need to feel that we shine above everything else in our caregiver's world – that we're the apple of their eye. Now, one might argue that some parts of modern society have taken this principle a little too far, but ultimately, it's a human need to feel that we matter in this way. Love isn't just about being one of many, it's about being witnessed and loved in our uniqueness and beauty.

Our Core Emotional Needs Are Connected

When one core emotional need isn't met, it will often impact the others. Indeed, there's a direct connection in the sense that we need boundaries to feel safe, and we need to feel safe to relax enough to feel love. Equally, a sense of love may be what gives us the confidence to hold a boundary or allows us to feel safe.

Furthermore, for many of us, our life is the result of the interplay between these different needs, and they're not being suitably met. In my own life, my sense that the world was unpredictable and dangerous, due to my sister's behavior, the lack of physical holding, and the lack of support in cultivating my strength due to the absence of my father, left me very vulnerable to being bullied at school.

I was normalized to violence and abuse, but I didn't have the strength necessary to stand up for myself. And my emotional neediness meant that on some level, I craved the attention that being bullied brought. In a perverse way, at least I was being seen and I felt special.

Now, of course, there are degrees with these emotional needs, and as we touched on in the last chapter, many of the struggles will be covert traumas. We don't need to be physically beaten to feel a lack of safety, and we don't need to be given abusive boundaries for our sense of strength to be diminished.

Were Your Core Emotional Needs Met?

To help increase your understanding of where you're currently at, let's explore which core emotional needs you did or didn't have met as a child. Answer the following questions using the worksheet in your free companion course at www.alexhoward.com/trauma.

Boundaries

- Were you given fair and reasonable boundaries that were held consistently?

- Were those boundaries sensitive and responsive to your needs, and were they adapted appropriately?

- Did you learn how to say no and was your 'no' respected?

- Were you challenged to take sensible risks and reach your potential?

- Were you allowed to struggle in healthy ways, and was self-discipline encouraged in response?

Safety

- Were you physically safe and protected as a child?

- Did you feel you had a 'soft place to fall,' emotionally?

- Were you given physical comfort and holding when you needed it?

- Did you feel that those around you were emotionally attuned to your feelings?

- Were your primary caregivers themselves in a calm and relaxed state most of the time, so you could relax into their safe holding?

Love

- Did you feel that your caregivers were interested in you and enjoyed spending time with you?

- Did your caregivers tell you they loved you?

- Did you feel love from your caregivers?

- Did you receive hugs, cuddles, and physical touch that was age-appropriate and made you feel loved?

- Were you made to feel that you were special to those around you?

What did you discover about yourself from completing this exercise? Did you get the boundaries, safety, and love that all children need? If not, that's OK. A key trajectory of our work together is for you to learn to meet these needs for yourself and increase your emotional resilience.

I recognize that you may have found the exercise difficult. For many of us, realizing that as children our fundamental needs were not met can be both shocking and deeply upsetting, as our heart longs for what we needed and deserved. If that's true for you, please be gentle with yourself.

Codependent Relationships

We'll talk more about the key relationships in our life in the final part of the book, but I'd like to point toward something specific now. When we feel a particular deficiency in an emotional need, we can unconsciously search for someone to meet that need in an intimate relationship.

For example, let's say we have poor boundaries and people walk all over us. As a result, we may find ourselves in a relationship with someone who's too strong and pushes through others' boundaries. On one level, there's a sense of relief for us in being with someone 'strong' who can protect us from other people, and even though they may disrespect and push through our own boundaries, there's also a strange familiarity in being related to in this way.

Ultimately, for our inner life and intimate relationships to work, we must learn to meet these needs inside ourselves. That's not to say that our intimate relationships can't help in supporting these needs, but they can't be the primary way that we meet them. Not having our core emotional needs met in childhood doesn't give us the best start in life, but we can learn to meet them for ourselves now, with practice and the right guidance.

Context in the ECHO Model

Bringing this all back to the ECHO way of thinking, the *context* within which the events of trauma happen is vitally important. How those around us, and we ourselves, respond to an event has a huge impact. Let's take the cases of two children who experience something as tragic as losing their mother.

In the first case, the family members are so consumed by their own sense of loss and grief that they pay little attention to the needs of the child. Indeed, seeing them upset may be too painful to witness and so they shout at them for crying. As a result, the child feels unsafe in their feelings and lacks a sense of adoration and care from those around them. They start acting out to get attention, and there are no boundaries that say, *we love you enough to say no.*

In the second case, the child isn't only given the physical and emotional holding they need, but they're also actively encouraged to have and to experience their emotions. When they feel sad, they're held in their tears, and the constant message is that they're loved and held. When they're caught acting out to get attention, they're given firm boundaries to adjust their behavior, but from a place of kindness and care.

Child one will likely go through life with a jacked-up nervous system through constantly running from how they feel, and all kinds of other negative outcomes resulting from their attempts to compensate for and avoid their pain.

Child two, as much as they'll deeply miss their mother, is held in the processing of their emotions and given the holding in their environment to limit the damage to many other areas of their life. Their pain isn't necessarily less at the time, but its impacts in their life are vastly different to child one's.

Unlock Your Future

I hope that by having read this chapter and completed the exercise you can now make more sense of how your childhood has shaped and challenged aspects of your adult life. More importantly, knowledge is power, and now that we're getting deeper into understanding what's shaped you, we can also go deeper into how to support healing.

And, as you're likely now realizing, the true damage of not getting our needs met in childhood isn't what happens in childhood, it's how it shapes us for the rest of our life. Ultimately, how we learn to relate to ourselves in our adult life is set up by these core emotional needs.

Our primary caregivers might not be around every day, but what we learn from them is. And until you deliberately change it, the chances are you're continuing to respond to yourself emotionally in the way that you were responded to. And that's exactly what we need to change. That's how we unlock your future from the limitations of your past.

Now it's time to get into the third of the four stages of trauma. In the next chapter we'll explore how our traumas affect the homeostatic balance of our nervous system, and the enormous impact this can have in our life.

CHAPTER 5

How's Your Homeostatic Balance?

When I first met Aadya she was in her early thirties and her most pressing symptom was intense migraines, which, according to her doctors, had no known cause. These were more than just bad headaches – they could last for three or four days and were so debilitating she had to lie in a darkened room until they passed.

At the point Aadya approached me, her migraines were being triggered almost weekly. Apart from the fact she was spending almost half her time trying to avoid any form of stimulation to survive this living hell, she was also starting to feel increasingly hopeless and depressed that things would never change.

I knew from Aadya's intake questionnaire that she'd experienced sustained physical abuse as a child, and it seemed plausible that there was a link between this and her migraines. As we explored her childhood together, she described some of the horrific events she'd endured, and I noticed that as she did so, there was a flatness and resignation to her expression and voice, and I had a strong sense that something inside of her had shut down in order to survive.

It was also obvious to me that Aadya was someone who lived in a state of high stress, and she was clearly experiencing anxiety, too. As I asked her about how she experienced her nervous system in her life now, she said that she certainly felt she was more easily triggered on a day-to-day basis than her friends were.

She often felt highly anxious about small things, and after a shock, it took her much longer than it should do for her system to recalibrate and settle back down into a state of calmness. In fact, even when she felt less wired, she noticed that there was an ongoing feeling of trepidation and a sense that the world was an unsafe place to be.

As Aadya continued to talk to me, what had happened in her body over the years became increasingly apparent. The abuse she'd suffered had been utterly overwhelming and would have been too much for anyone, let alone a child, to process. Unable to leave the unsafe environment physically, Aadya did the next best thing – she left it emotionally and retreated to her mind.

A Maladaptive Stress Response

Part of the genius of the human organism is that when we face the threat of danger, our nervous system switches gears to protect us. In Aadya's case, this meant her system had become hyper-activated and sensitized to any kind of threat. This speeding up of the nervous system serves a dual purpose – it prepares us for immediate danger and it also allows us to disconnect from the resultant difficult feelings that we don't feel safe to process.[1]

Aadya's body's response hadn't just been the best option available to her, it'd been the reason she'd survived. However, her survival had come at a price. Her nervous system had become normalized to living in a constant state of stress, and she was so familiar with being this way that she barely noticed it. That was, until the migraines became so intense that she'd no choice but to look for help.

I explained to Aadya that her migraines were not in themselves the issue – they were a symptom of an underlying issue, which was that her nervous system was dysregulated (impaired and not functioning in the way it should be). Aadya was living in what I'd many years earlier come to call a maladaptive stress response. As is so often the case, the impact of her trauma wasn't ultimately in the original event, but in the changes in her stress response and the outcomes in her life. To understand Aadya's experience further, let's look at the mechanics of what happens in the body when the stress response is triggered.

Fight, Freeze, Flight

Imagine that you and I are walking down the street when we suddenly spot a huge electric bus heading straight for us. In that moment of frantic realization that our time on Earth might be coming to a swift and messy end, we can choose to respond in one of three ways:

- **Fight** – I think we both know that won't end well, as buses don't break easily!

- **Freeze** – Again, this isn't my preferred choice in this instance.

- **Flight** – We can run as fast as possible to the pavement.

When it comes to meeting threat in our lives, each of these responses has been painstakingly tested through millions of years of evolution. Sometimes, fighting is the best way to survive; other times freezing and hoping that we haven't been seen is our saving grace; and other times still, we need to flee as fast as our legs will carry us.

Now, whichever response we choose, it's going to be labor-intensive, so we need the resources to do so. When our nervous system is triggered into a stress response, almost immediately our heart rate increases and blood starts flowing away from non-survival-based functions, such as digestion, to our arms and legs, allowing us to leap into action. Alongside this, our adrenal glands release more of the hormones adrenaline and cortisol to fuel our body.

At the same time, our emotional center shuts down because exploring the nuanced and complex emotions we have about the situation – for example, how it reminds us of being dominated by an overbearing parent – holds no value for our immediate survival.

Freezing our emotions is a sensible way to survive that moment, but it has a huge price in the long term. For a compelling exploration of the health consequences of long-term emotional shut down or disconnection, I recommend Dr. Gabor Maté's excellent book *When the Body Says No*.[2]

The Power of the Unconscious Mind

The American writer Mark Twain famously said: 'I've seen many troubles in my time, only half of which ever came true.' The truth, though, is even more tragic. You see, as I mentioned earlier, research shows that our unconscious mind can't tell the difference between something that's real and something that's vividly imagined.

Here's an example of this. I'd like you to close your eyes and imagine that in your left hand you're holding a ripe, juicy lemon. Move the lemon close to your nose and smell its fresh aroma. Now imagine that you're holding a knife in your right hand and are carefully cutting the lemon in half. Hold one half of the lemon close to your nose and once again smell it, noticing how much stronger the aroma has become. Next, I'd like you to move the lemon toward your mouth and take a large bite out of it.

What happened as you imagined doing this? Did you start to produce saliva, and perhaps have a strong, visceral response to biting the lemon?

Here's the thing – you were simply imagining something, but your body responded as if it were real.

Now let's look at how this works with our stress response. Just as we can imagine eating a lemon and our body responds as though it's real, our stress response doesn't need actual, real physical danger to be triggered. Indeed, for the majority of us, for most of the time, what's triggering our stress response is *imagined* danger.

To add to the problem, research demonstrates that when we're activated in a stress response, we're more likely to perceive a non-threatening situation as dangerous.[3,4] In a sense, we have a confirmation bias in that we look for danger and threat and we find it, even when it isn't there. So, once we get used to being in a stress response, in a way, it becomes self-generating.

System Overload

Furthermore, our body's stress response is designed to be used to respond to acute and short-term stressors. What it isn't designed for is the kind of ongoing, chronic stress that many of us experience in our daily lives these days.

From the moment we wake up to the moment we go to bed, we experience micro triggers everywhere – from social media and the 24-hour news cycle to the frantic pace of modern life and the stressful commute to and from work. In time, our nervous system becomes overloaded by the constant demands placed on it, which is why there's so much research demonstrating the relationship between chronic stress and everything from chronic pain to sleep issues, anxiety, depression, and chronic fatigue.[5-10]

What Is Homeostatic Balance?

Now, as interesting as all this is, there's a crucially important piece in how this helps us understand the four stages, or ECHOs, of trauma. You see, when we consistently trigger our stress response, our body starts to learn that this is normal, and so it adapts to it becoming our baseline, or our new homeostatic balance.[11,12]

The body has all kinds of homeostatic balances, from blood pressure and temperature to the circadian rhythms that manage our hormone levels based on our regular sleep and awake times. The term homeostasis is derived from two Greek words meaning 'same' and 'stable,' and in a sense, our homeostatic balances are the body's way of keeping things the same and stable, to support consistent and reliable ongoing functioning.

Our homeostatic balance allows us to feel safe and steady and is heavily influenced by whatever state we live in as our normal. The problem, though, is that repeated exposure to trauma triggers, and our inability to regulate our nervous system, leads our homeostatic balance to shift.

Over time, our body adapts and normalizes to a state of high stress, and it works to maintain and sustain this level as normal. This is a maladaptive stress response – a stress response that's normalized to an abnormal level of high alert and so has become maladaptive.

The result is that our body is now working to maintain a level of stress. Indeed, in the short term if we try to calm our system, as soon as we stop, it'll return to the higher level of arousal that it's learned is normal. When we experience ongoing stress as a child, ultimately, we're training a shift in our homeostatic balance that can define our life as an adult.[13-16]

It's also worth noting that the danger of living in this way is that it becomes a self-fulfilling prophecy. We learn that safety is a product of being in this maladaptive stress response, because despite the price we pay to do so, we notice that we do survive the bumps and scrapes of our life, and our system learns that this must be the result of the state we're living in, regardless of whether this is true or not. It might be deeply uncomfortable, but our unconscious believes that it works.

And so, the more anxiety we have, the more justified and intense our stress response becomes. Like a self-generating power source, the more anxious we become, the more entrenched we become in this response.

A Maladaptive Stress Response and Our Physical Body

The impact of sustained stress on our physical body – from our immune system to our digestive system, and from our hormones to our nervous system – is very well documented in modern science. For example, the field of psychoneuroimmunology (PNI) has established that psychological stress disrupts the interaction between the nervous and immune systems.

Stress-induced immune dysregulation has been shown to be significant enough to result in health consequences, including reducing the immune response to vaccines, slowing wound healing, reactivating latent herpes viruses, such as Epstein–Barr virus (EBV), and increasing the risk for more severe infectious disease.[17–20]

A Maladaptive Stress Response and Our Emotional Body

When our emotional body is functioning naturally and healthily, we're able to process our emotions in a way that's similar to how our digestive system processes food. There are four stages to this:

- Chewing – just as we do with food, we chew on our emotions. This is where we talk about and sit with things, and they break down a little and become more manageable.

- Digesting – just as our stomach breaks down food, our emotional body starts to tease apart our emotions and begin the process of working through them. We allow ourselves to actually feel our emotions. This might be a bit intense at first, but if we stay with the experience, our emotions move and evolve.

- Absorbing – our small intestine extracts the goodness, or nutrients, from our food, and we do the same with our emotions. We take the learnings and they feed and nurture us, even when we experience painful emotions.

- Expelling – when the goodness has been extracted from our food, we'll excrete the waste products. The same is true with our emotions – once we've absorbed what we need to, it's time to expel and move on.

A problem occurs when this process is unable to work properly. Just as stress will cause digestive issues in our physical body, when we go into a maladaptive stress response, we become unable to process our emotions and they get stuck in our emotional body.

How a Maladaptive Stress Response Blocks Healing

In my work with chronic illnesses, one of the phrases I use most often is, 'For our body to heal, it has to be in a healing state.' In this context, I'm referring to our physical body, but the same is true of our emotional body. When we're in a maladaptive stress response, we're blocked to the very healing that we need. To open to, digest, and metabolize our emotions, we must first learn to calm and reset our nervous system.

Furthermore, the feeling of safety we're so deeply seeking simply cannot be found when our body's pumped full of stress hormones, our mind is running at twice the speed it needs to, and we're locked in a state of constant tension. Ultimately, safety is a feeling that exists in our body, not as a state in our nervous system and mind. And because safety is a feeling, you can't *think* your way to a *feeling* of safety. Please read that again: You can't THINK your way to a FEELING of safety.

The Safety Loop

Let's return to Aadya's story for a moment. The reason why she felt so painfully stuck was because all the known ways out of her anxiety involved thinking harder and faster, and the more she did so, the more likely she was to have a migraine.

As everyone does when in this state, Aadya had tried thinking through every possible outcome and scenario, and as a bright young woman, she'd come up with many. This dilemma is what I call the safety loop. The more we feel unsafe, the more our mind and nervous system speed up to try and protect us; the more we disconnect from our body and get lost in the realms of our mind, the more unsafe we end up feeling. And the further away we become from the very feeling of safety that we need.

To build the feeling of safety in our body, we must learn to switch off our maladaptive stress response, reset our homeostatic balances, and train our nervous system into a healing state. With a calmer nervous system, we'll then find the *feeling* of safety that we seek in our body.

Are You Living in a Maladaptive Stress Response?

To help lay the foundations for resetting your nervous system, I'd like to spend a little time exploring its current state. Remember, the point of this is to start to create healing and change, and knowledge can help us do so. Think about the following questions and then respond to them using the worksheet at www.alexhoward.com/trauma.

- Do you often feel 'wired' and as if you can't relax?

- Do you have difficulty sleeping?

- When you do manage to relax, do you often feel exhausted?

- Does your mind race?

- Do you find yourself constantly replaying conversations in your mind?

- Do you spend a lot of time thinking about possible future scenarios?

- Do you feel drained while you're around other people?

If you've answered yes to any of these questions, then there's a good chance your nervous system needs some help to calm and reset. You may also notice that at different points in the day it's more agitated than others, and that around particular people and situations you're much more easily triggered.

Change Is Possible

As Aadya worked with me using the RESET model we'll explore later, she was able to reset her homeostatic balance, and almost immediately she noticed a reduction in the frequency and intensity of her migraines. As we then worked to bring into balance the 'perfectionist' and 'achiever' patterns that had become her strategies to try and win love (you'll learn about these personality patterns in Chapter 8), her migraines stopped happening almost completely.

And this is our next focus: understanding the strategies that you've developed in your life to attempt to manage the outcomes of your trauma.

CHAPTER 6

The Outcomes of
Your Trauma

When I first met Fergus, he was in his late twenties and battling chronic fatigue syndrome (CFS). A likeable guy with a quiet charm and a lively sense of humor, he was using his strong intellect to dive deep into the biomedical aspects of fatigue and working hard to find a path to recovery.

Not wanting to leave any stone unturned, Fergus had started working with me on the psychology side of his healing. Although he was certain that his illness was in his body and not his mind, his research had demonstrated that the mind, emotions, and body are deeply connected.

From our first session, it was obvious to me that Fergus was out of touch with himself emotionally. He could easily engage with practical exercises to grow awareness of his thoughts, and things that involved willpower or effort were no issue for him. But, when it came to slowing down and connecting emotionally, I might as well have been asking him to solve Pythagorean Theorem.

As we'll explore later, there are different defenses and strategies we use to train ourselves to not feel our emotions. For Fergus, this looked like always being busy and using his mind as a way of analyzing and distancing himself from how he felt. Although his intellect was a valuable tool in his day-to-day life, it was in danger of becoming a major block to connecting to his heart and emotions.

Emotional Freezing

Wishing to understand more deeply the origins of Fergus's emotional shutdown, in one session I questioned him about his childhood and what he'd been taught about his feelings. He told me that at the age of eight he'd been sent to one of the UK's top boarding schools, frequented by British royalty and the upper echelons of society.

Fergus didn't come from a particularly wealthy family, so the school fees alone had been the source of considerable financial strain for his parents. But it was a burden they were willing to bear because their children were the most important thing in their lives, and they wanted to give them the very best start possible.

For Fergus's parents, sending their son to boarding school was an act of love, but he experienced it as the ultimate rejection. Beyond the fact that eight is a very young age for a child to be separated from their parents for months on end, Fergus was also a particularly sensitive boy. During his first weeks at the school, he cried himself to sleep every night, longing for his mother's comfort and reassurance. Ultimately, he was craving the emotional need for love.

This was in the days before mobile phones and email, and the only means of communication the children were allowed was a letter every few weeks. Fergus counted the days until he could write his first letter, convinced that once his mother realized just how unhappy he was she'd let him come home.

However, what he didn't know was that the letters were vetted before being sent, and the following day he was taken aside by his housemaster and instructed to rewrite his letter as the contents might be too upsetting for his mother to read. With his only lifeline to the comfort that he so desperately craved cut off, Fergus realized he had a choice – he could continue to cry himself to sleep every night and live in the emotional hell his life had become, or he could shut down his emotions; he opted for the latter.

The teachers at Fergus's school strongly promoted the virtues of being 'tough' and not showing emotion; part of the generation who'd grown up in postwar Britain, they valued keeping a 'stiff upper lip,' and if Fergus was going to survive, he had to follow their lead. Put another way, they taught him the wrong kind of strength, and he learned that it was no longer safe to show his emotions.

The more Fergus shut down his emotions and vulnerability, the more he thrived in school life, and by the time the holidays finally came he was highly practiced at it and felt a sense of pride at showing his parents how 'strong' he'd become. He was on the way to becoming an emotionally disconnected man before his age hit double digits.

And the more Fergus disconnected from his emotions, the more he learned to live in his mind as a place of comfort. He learned that emotions are a sign of weakness; that thoughts are better than emotions; and that if he fell apart emotionally, no one would be there to hold him.

Fergus performed well academically, and he continued to develop his intellectual reasoning skills over his emotional sensitivity. The only hint of the emotional pain he'd buried was his aggression on the rugby field, the sport being a blessed outlet for his anger and hurt.

How Our Defenses Become Our Prison

As Fergus relayed this story, he showed barely a hint of emotion; he might have been talking about someone else's life. On some level, he knew that what he was revealing was significant, but he was almost completely disconnected from the emotional impact of the life he was describing.

The more Fergus talked, the clearer it became that retreating into his mind had been a defense against his true feelings and emotions. The problem was that the fortress he'd built around his heart had now become a prison. The walls he'd built to help keep the world out were keeping him trapped inside.

Furthermore, we cannot close our heart selectively. If we allow ourselves to feel love, we risk feeling loss. So, by closing his heart to his pain, longing, and sadness, Fergus was also closing his heart to love, joy, and the capacity to feel emotional connection to others. The consequence was that long before he'd had issues with his health, Fergus had struggled with emotional intimacy, particularly in relationships. He pushed people away, and was unable to be vulnerable, and the result was that although he longed to be in a long-term relationship, he seemed to lack the capacity to do so.

Let's look at Fergus's situation in the context of the four stages, or ECHOs, of trauma. As a child, he'd suffered the traumatic event of being separated from his parents before he was ready, and the separation itself meant he was cut off from the very love he needed. Furthermore, Fergus had become used to the fact that he had a constant background feeling of anxiety and the sense that the world wasn't a safe place – i.e., his homeostatic balance had shifted.

However, what was most damaging for Fergus wasn't so much the event, but the *beliefs* and *behaviors* he'd learned from the experience, which, going forward, had echoed throughout every area of his life. When we learn that our emotions aren't safe, and that they're not welcome, these are not just beliefs that get set up for the short term – instead, they become our operating system for life.

Of course, we don't come up with these beliefs in isolation; they're often heavily influenced by the environment around us, which is far from helped by the medical professionals that many of us look to for guidance. To help you make sense of this, please indulge me while I share a brief overview of the roots of modern psychology...

A Brief History of Modern Psychology

Most experts credit the inception of the field of psychology as we know it to the American philosopher William James in the late 19th century. Although James's work was truly groundbreaking at the time, it was his view that emotion is the result of our mind's perception of our environment. Put another way, emotion is a product of our thinking mind, not a living entity in itself, with its own wisdom and sensitivities.

A few decades later, along came the great Sigmund Freud, an Austrian neurologist who founded psychoanalytic theory. Although Freud, too, made some hugely important contributions to our understanding of the human condition, in psychoanalysis, he saw emotions as a byproduct of our unruly unconscious mind. They're something to be suspicious of, rather than nurtured and opened to.

In response to Freud's preoccupation with the unruly and untrainable world of the unconscious, a more pragmatic psychological approach took hold in the mid-1950s with the model of behavioral psychology. Inspired by Pavlov's famous experiments on his unfortunate dogs 50 years earlier, behavioral psychologists attempted to reduce the human condition to our predictable and trainable reactions to the complex world around us.

In the 1960s, the realization that the world we inhabit is not that simple gave rise to cognitive psychology. Cognitive psychologists made the rather fundamental point that two people can be exposed to the same stimulus and yet demonstrate a very different response. They focused on what they called the mysterious 'black box' between stimulus and response and attempted to explain human experience by our logical thinking processes.

And then, in the 1980s, a seeming miracle occurred in the world of academic psychology when the enemy camps of behavioral psychology and cognitive psychology took a proverbial deep breath and realized that perhaps they might *both* be right. Cognitive behavioral therapy (CBT) was born, and it's been the mainstream psychological approach ever since. CBT is primarily about using rational thinking to change our thoughts and behaviors and has little time for feelings and emotions.

Relegating the Heart

Now, although I certainly believe that CBT has its place, the hugely disproportionate amount of research money it's received compared to many other psychological approaches has simply served to build the assumption that it's the only effective approach. And CBT also misses a fundamental point – human beings are so much more than their mind.

The word 'psychology' is derived from the Greek word 'psyche,' which means 'life' or 'breath.' Some other derived meanings of the word include 'self' or 'soul.' My preferred definition is that psychology is ultimately the study of the soul. That being the case, the excellent progress that traditional psychology has made in studying the arena of the mind has missed the fact that our mind is just a small part of our ultimate experience. How about our heart? Our feelings? Our emotions? Can these all just be reduced to our rational (or indeed irrational) cognitions about the world around us?

Of course, it makes sense that traditional psychology focuses in the way it does – it's a product of academic institutions that value intellect, reasoning, and logic above all else. In more recent years the American Psychiatric Association's *Diagnostic and Statistical Manual of Mental Disorders* (DSM-V) has been criticized for having been influenced by the pharmaceutical industry,[1,2] for pathologizing healthy reactions to life events, and for being culturally insensitive to the experiences of women and of people from marginalized cultures.[3,4]

In fact, you might be shocked to hear that the third iteration of the DSM in the 1970s (upon which later editions are still based) was produced by a very small group of white male psychiatrists who held a series of meetings and took votes on what they considered 'normal'.[5] It was very far from being a truly scientific and inclusive or culturally representative process.

Indeed, when was the last time you heard someone speak of the longings and wishes of the heart in a university lecture theater? In the years I spent studying psychology, the closest a lecturer came to exploring emotions was when describing the various signs of paranoia and mental illness.

Toxic Positivity

It's not only the field of psychology that's contributed to a relegation of the heart and emotions to a minor footnote in the story of our lives – much of the popular psychology movement has followed a somewhat similar tack. Often, emotions are divided into categories of 'positive' and 'negative.' So, the goal becomes, how can we experience more positive emotions, such as happiness and excitement, and fewer negative emotions, such as sadness and anxiety?

As we'll discuss later, in truth, all emotions are 'positive' because they all have something important to communicate to us and deserve to be witnessed and experienced. The constant prioritizing of 'positive' emotions tends to go alongside a general attitude of 'just look for the positive' or 'good vibes only.' In some circles, this has come to be called toxic positivity, and I think, rightly so – just as junk food damages our physical body, so toxic positivity can damage our emotional body.

I'm not suggesting that we should wallow in our emotions and become stuck in them; however, they do need to be allowed to move through us, in the way I described in the last chapter, and the rejection of large parts of our emotional range ends up causing a world of pain for us and quite possibly those around us.

Emotional Suppression

At this point, though, you'd be forgiven for thinking, how on earth is it possible for large parts of society to simply ignore the callings of their heart – to effectively assign their emotional life to an eternal purgatory?

Well, in reality, what happens is that the emotions don't evaporate or disappear (if only life was that simple.) Instead, they're suppressed into our unconscious, which means they're a living part of our experience but we're unable to connect with them or understand them.

As we touched on in Chapter 2, we all walk around with a metaphorical black sack containing all the traumas and emotions we've experienced but not processed and digested. If everything's going to plan in our life and we're not exposed to further shocks or traumas, we might be able to function relatively easily (or at least appear to on the surface). But when we get pushed beyond our coping limits, or we experience a shock, the top of that black sack opens, and we experience an explosion of unprocessed traumas and emotions. And then, once we've let off steam, the chances are the top gets tightly sealed again.

The more we suppress our emotions, and the deeper we push them away, the more dangerous they become in our life – like a toxic substance that festers and eats away at everything we value as important.

Sometimes, unprocessed emotional pain expresses itself as physical pain. Indeed, there's a growing body of evidence demonstrating the relationship between chronic pain and childhood trauma, for example.[6-10] When we don't process our emotional pain as a child, it's held in our body as physical pain in our future. Some people experience their emotional disconnection in the anxiety that comes from living in their mind.

And the more our emotions are rejected, the more they color the lens through which we see the world around us. Indeed, we don't see the world as it really is – we see it through the lens of our beliefs and the meanings we've created.[11] To truly heal the emotional impacts of our trauma, we must first understand the beliefs and meanings that obscure our ability to see ourselves and the world clearly.

The Impact of Our Beliefs

It's thought that in any given moment, our conscious mind can work with around seven pieces of information.[12,13] For example, right now, my mind is focusing on the words I'm writing and how they fit the focus of the chapter; I'm aware of my dogs sleeping next to me in their basket (and one of them snoring!); I can feel some inner pressure to hit my target wordcount for the day; and I'm listening to rock music louder than I probably should.

In this moment, there are lots of things going on that I could be aware of but I'm not – such as the changing light and cooling temperature as evening falls outside, and the stiffness in my lower back from sitting all day.

In fact, it's estimated that every second, we receive about 11 million pieces of information from our senses.[14] Forty or fifty of those are captured by our brain, and just seven can be held and processed by our working memory at any one time. To manage the compression needed to achieve this, our brain uses mental shortcuts, and these can often unconsciously lead to poor decisions or cognitive bias (which is where we see a limited data set that's influenced by our perspective).[15-17]

So, with our conscious mind having bandwidth for just seven things, we need to be able to prioritize what we focus on, and that's the service that our beliefs provide for us – they give us a critical shortcut. Our beliefs are like a map that helps us navigate the complex and overwhelming world around us.

Here's an example of how beliefs develop. When we're small and learning to walk, we'll soon encounter the wonder that is the door. At first, doors will seem like a magical mystery – sometimes they're open, other times they're closed. We then discover that we can push or pull to open and close them. However, once we've learned how doors open, we've learned doors, and we can then use them.

As time passes, we'll come to realize that sometimes doors are locked, and we need the key. Eventually, we'll figure out sliding doors versus doors on hinges. But, each time we learn, we update and develop our internal learning of doors, and if you'll excuse a cliché, that will open lots of doors for us.

Emotional Groundhog Day

Let's look at this in the context of Fergus's story. As a child, he had intense emotional pain that he was actively told he wasn't allowed to feel, and so to survive a highly distressing emotional experience, he learned to shut off his feelings. He took on the belief in his environment that *feeling your emotions is dangerous and weak,* and from that moment on, it became the lens through which he perceived the world.

Notice that Fergus didn't learn a more nuanced belief, such as, *If you want to survive at a stiff-upper-lip English boarding school, you need to shut down your emotions. However, ultimately, your feelings are both hugely important and totally valid, and the problem lies with the environment, not you.* Indeed, if he had, the impact would have been much less.

As we've touched on a few times, the real trauma of the event wasn't the event itself, it was the programming setup in Fergus which, 20 years later, was causing deep misery and suffering in many different areas of his life. Because of the beliefs Fergus had learned, he was living in an emotional Groundhog Day, recreating his own trauma for himself day after day.

The Two Types of Beliefs

Beliefs can be put into two distinct categories. The first is consequential beliefs, which are those where we assume that one thing is the result of another. Examples include: 'If I show my emotions, people will reject me' and 'If I ask for help, people will laugh at me.' The second category is global beliefs, which are generalized beliefs about the world around us (remember our need to simplify the world from 11 million pieces of information to seven.) Examples include 'Most people are bad' or 'The world's a scary place.'

Each of us holds numerous consequential and global beliefs about ourselves, our feelings, other people, and the world around us. Now, not all beliefs are wrong, and some of them might be relatively accurate. However, until we go through a careful process of examining and reflecting on these beliefs, we've no idea which are which, because the reality is they were shaped impulsively in response to overwhelming and complex situations that we didn't understand at the time.

To begin the process of loosening the grip of some of your beliefs, we must identify what they are in the first place. A phrase I often use is, 'If you can see it, you don't have to be it.' Put another way, the very naming of a belief will often begin a process of questioning it in our mind, which can help us make a conscious choice about whether we want to continue to relate to ourselves and the world around us through this lens.

What Do You Believe About Your Emotions?

Having explored the enormous impact that our beliefs have, it's time to delve into some of your beliefs. So, what do you believe about emotions and their place in your world? Write down at least three consequential and three global beliefs that you identify with. To help you, I've given a few examples of common beliefs of both types that people hold. You may find that some of these feel true to you, or you might find that you discover different beliefs.

Consequential Beliefs

- If I feel my emotions, I'll fall apart.
- If I'm vulnerable, people will take advantage of me.
- If I ask for what I need, I'll get hurt.

Global Beliefs

- Emotions are a sign of weakness.
- People are inherently selfish.
- All men/women/people are cruel and want to hurt you.
- Logic is superior to emotions.

Once again, if you find yourself feeling shocked and more vulnerable after seeing what you've written in response to these questions, please be gentle with yourself. We'll be looking at ways to change and challenge these beliefs later.

How Our Beliefs Become Our Personality

As we gradually develop various beliefs about ourselves and the world around us through childhood and beyond, we're effectively setting up and programming our default ways of being and responding in the world.

Perhaps we learn that being loved by others is a result of what we achieve in the world, and so being a high achiever becomes our core focus in life. Or perhaps the conclusion we draw from childhood is that the secret to being safe is to be in control of everything and everyone around us, and so a constant need for control starts seeping into every part of our life.

In a sense, clusters of beliefs start forming the core ways that we relate to ourselves and the world around us. In Chapter 8 we'll look at some of the key personality patterns that can perpetuate our cycles of trauma. First though, it's time to explore the RESET model for healing the impacts of your trauma.

PART II

The RESET Solution for Trauma Healing

INTRODUCTION

In Part I we explored the ECHO model for understanding the origins of your trauma. My hope is that this has helped you make sense of yourself and your history in a new way. In this part of the book, we'll be looking at the RESET model for healing the impacts of your trauma by resetting your nervous system.

The RESET model has been at the core of my work with trauma in its many forms over the past two decades. It was shaped both by the enormous laboratory of learnings that have come from the dozens of practitioners at The Optimum Health Clinic working with thousands of patients, and by the hundreds of graduates that have come through our Therapeutic Coaching® practitioner training and the thousands of people that they've worked with.

The RESET model has been carefully designed to ensure that its tools and strategies are sequenced in the correct order. For example, before we work on processing and healing your trauma, we first need to make sure that you have the right foundations in place. Each step in the RESET sequence is important and skipping steps often slows down rather than speeds up the healing journey.

Indeed, one of the most common things people say when they go through my online RESET Program® is that they finally understand how previous interventions had made things worse rather than better and that they now need to sequence their healing to ensure that it works.

Five Steps to RESET Your Nervous System

Here's an overview of the five steps of the RESET model: we'll look at these in depth in the coming chapters:

1: Recognize

Which state is your nervous system in?
Remember what I said earlier, 'If you can see it, you don't have to be it.' To work to reset your nervous system, we must first make you aware of the state it's in right now. Both on the macro level of recognizing if your nervous system is dysregulated, and on the micro level of being aware of what's happening with it day-to-day and moment-to-moment.

2: Examine

How is this state being created?
Once you've recognized which state your nervous system's in right now, we need to dig deeper to understand the personality patterns, thinking, and behaviors that are driving and maintaining this state. You've already done a certain amount of work on this in Part I, but by bringing things together in specific ways, we can start being targeted about changing these patterns.

3: Stop

Rewire your brain and prevent unhelpful thought patterns.
Two things need to happen at this stage. The first is learning to retrain your nervous system through practices such as meditation. The second is actively

stopping the momentum of the patterns of thinking and behavior that are maintaining your maladaptive stress response. By habitually resetting your homeostatic balance, in time it will start to shift to a calmer state.

4: Emotions

Connect to and process your emotions.

With trauma, one of the reasons our nervous system becomes activated is to help us escape the overwhelming emotions that we don't have the support and resources to process. As we start to retrain our nervous system into a calmer place, we can find ourselves re-experiencing some of these emotions, and so having the tools and strategies to help us process them is an important part of our deeper healing. Furthermore, it's this healing that allows us to stay connected to our body and emotions in a healthy and sustainable way.

5: Transform

Change your relationship with yourself.

As we continue to process our emotions, we now have the potential for a fundamental shift in the way we relate to ourselves and the world around us. Remember the three core emotional needs that affect the context of how events impact us – developing an inner sense of boundaries, safety, and love is critical not only for healing the past but also for increasing our emotional resilience in the future.

A Final Note

Before we jump into the RESET model, there's one more thing I'd like to point out. If you were working with us one-to-one in the clinic, or through one of my self-led or group programs, we'd be constantly reminding you to not just listen to but to truly honor your own lived experience. This is even more important when your experience tells you something different to what I do in the book.

The RESET model is a framework. It's not perfect, and everyone's lived experience is unique to them. So, please listen to your own inner guidance, and know that the act of tuning in and responding to your experience is in itself a healing practice. Put another way: I know that my RESET model is helpful to a lot of people, but your lived experience matters more.

CHAPTER 7

Recognize Which State Your Nervous System Is In

When I was a child, the word anxiety wasn't in my vocabulary – not because I wasn't anxious, but because, a bit like an Inuit who's never known a balmy summer's day, I just assumed that the way I felt was how other people felt too.

As I look back at my younger self today, I can see many signs of the hyped-up state within which my nervous system lived. Apart from the physical impacts of irritable bowel syndrome and in time, the chronic illness ME/CFS, my emotional state was also a constant challenge. I was hypersensitive emotionally – overly merging with others' feelings – and searching for physical and emotional safety was far more of a focus day-to-day than it should have been. Anxiety wasn't just a state that I sometimes found myself in, but the emotional home I'd normalized to.

Although I might have adapted to the way I felt, there were obvious clues on the surface that my nervous system was running too fast. I ate my food too fast, my mind ran too fast, and I moved too fast. Most notably to others, I also spoke very quickly – for much of my childhood people would constantly ask me to speak more slowly and to stop mumbling. Alas, it did little to help, because of course, for most of us, the way we use our voice isn't something we tend to consciously modulate and control; instead, it just reflects the state we're in.

Why Awareness Is Key

As part of growing my training and experience as a therapist, I did several courses in hypnotherapy. And as I discovered just how important our voice is for intentional communication – which of course is at the heart of any kind of effective therapeutic work – learning to slow down my voice became one of my key focuses.

A few months into one hypnotherapy training course, we were encouraged to practice recording guided meditation and hypnosis sessions – firstly to get used to how our voice sounded, but also to gather feedback from others about how we could improve. Feeling optimistic that my efforts had paid off and that my voice would now be the therapeutic tool I hoped for, I cracked on with my homework.

However, my reaction on hearing the recordings I made was a rather painful and awkward silence. I'd deliberately slowed my voice to what I thought was a calming and soothing pace, but it was still significantly faster than the average person's speaking voice. I had to halve the speed at which I spoke, and then halve it again to sound even vaguely relaxing.

Early on in my work at The Optimum Health Clinic, I realized that my experience was far from unique – in fact, it was very common. Many of the people I was working with to calm their maladaptive stress response had no idea just how dysregulated their nervous system was. Even if they knew intellectually that they were not in a calm state, the consistency and intensity of their nervous system's over-arousal was still outside their conscious awareness.

Remember, part of the brilliant design of the human system is our ability to normalize to whatever becomes our consistent experience. And so, to be truly effective in learning to reset our nervous system, we must first become aware of the state it's in. I'll say it again: If you can *see* it, you don't have to *be* it.

In Chapter 5 we began to look at how being in a maladaptive stress response will impact on our physical, mental, and emotional health. In this chapter, we're going to focus on learning to truly *recognize* when your body is in a state of maladaptive stress response and then understand what's triggering it.

The Three States of the Nervous System

When it comes to understanding the states of our nervous system, the work of Dr. Stephen Porges, a professor of psychiatry at the University of North Carolina in the USA, is immensely helpful. Professor Porges's work has become known as Polyvagal Theory (poly = many; vagal = wandering).

Originally, Porges had been researching the vagus nerve, which connects our brain with our digestion and other bodily systems. He came to realize that there was a fundamental gap in the research into stress, which focused on the activated stress response via the sympathetic nervous system, a branch of the autonomic nervous system.

However, this activated stress response didn't match the lived experience of many of those living with trauma. Indeed, for trauma victims a more common experience is feeling shut down and immobilized, and this often makes them more susceptible to further negative experiences because their ability to defend and fight for themselves isn't activated.

Put another way, we can be in a stress state without being in the fight or flight state we discussed in Chapter 5. In fact, sometimes our most activated state of stress is a state of freeze or shut-down. The effects of unprocessed trauma, along with ideas about releasing them, are described in the seminal work *The Body Keeps the Score* by Bessel van der Kolk.[1]

Professor Porges went on to study the parasympathetic nervous system, another part of the autonomic nervous system. The primary nerve of the parasympathetic nervous system is the vagus, which has two pathways originating from different areas of the brainstem – the dorsal pathway and the ventral pathway.

The dorsal vagus is evolutionarily older and is shared with most vertebrates. However, the functioning of the ventral pathway, which is to calm us and connect us socially, is limited to mammals. Professor Porges documented that the more primitive dorsal vagus is responsible for our nervous system shutting down or 'freezing.'

According to Porges, there are three states that our nervous system can be in: socialization, mobilization, and immobilization. Let's explore these now.

1: Socialization

Polyvagal Theory highlights that human beings are social animals and that our nervous system is wired to relax through positive human interaction. Just as babies relax through co-regulating their nervous system with those of their caregivers, as adults we're wired to look for safety cues from those around us. In a sense, nourishing contact with other people is more than just a nice experience – it's a key building block for being in a healing state and sending the message to our nervous system to relax because we're safe.

When we have positive and supportive experiences with our primary caregivers as children, it not only helps soothe our developing nervous system, but it also sets up a positive foundation for our relationships going forward. Furthermore, it also teaches our nervous system how to self-regulate, and so we can self-soothe when we're alone.

Ultimately, when our socialization system is activated, we're in a healing state. This means we can relax deeply, respond appropriately to the world around us, and if we have emotional healing work to do, we're able to do it.

2: Mobilization

In this state, we're ready for action and instinctively prepared to deal with danger. We can do this by fighting it or fleeing (running away from it). In an acute state of fight or flight, we may be aware of stress hormones such as adrenaline and cortisol flooding through our system because we'll feel primed, or mobilized, for action. Depending on the nature of the situation, emotionally we might feel excited and energized if the stress is positive and fearful and in danger if it's not.

When we're in a chronic state of fight or flight (as in the experience I described at the start of the chapter), we'll likely have normalized to the state we're in. What's particularly problematic about this is that the negative impacts on our body are there but we're unaware of the state that's driving them. This is when the awareness we've been talking about is so important because it allows us to work to calm this response.

3. Immobilization

When an animal is under extreme threat, sometimes fighting with or running away from the threat is ineffective or likely to make the situation worse. For example, imagine a rabbit pottering around when it suddenly spots a wolf in the distance. The rabbit has no chance of winning in a fight with the wolf, and although it might win the race if it flees, it's a risky move. So instead, it reflexively collapses and appears to be dead, showing itself as of no interest or threat to the wolf, and indeed hoping it doesn't even notice it. For the rabbit, freezing and immobilizing itself is the best survival response it has.

Years ago, I saw a live TV show in which a small child, when asked a question by the host, froze, and appeared to almost stop breathing. The host tried multiple ways to get a response, all to no avail – the child had frozen as a form of self-protection, until the spotlight was off them and they could relax again.

Sometimes our nervous system will go into a freeze response because it's the best option; other times it will do it because of an overload of mobilization. It's almost as if our system blows a fuse and shuts down in an attempt to protect itself from further threat and danger.

However, despite the lack of movement, there's often a great deal of energy tied up in sustaining immobilization. What can appear, on the surface, to be a state devoid of energy is in fact one of intense energy *demand*, which will drain our already depleted system further still.

Know Your Baseline

As you may have noticed, there's a sequence to these three states of the nervous system. A healing state of socialization is a healthy baseline for the nervous system; however, if we're triggered into stress, our baseline is raised and we progress to mobilization, which, at its extreme, can turn to immobilization.

Returning to our ECHO model, remember that one of the major impacts of trauma is that it shifts our homeostatic balance, ultimately affecting the baseline to which our nervous system returns. A key part of the work we're doing in this book is retraining your baseline back to socialization and a normal level of functioning.

When it comes to understanding your nervous system, you don't just need to be aware of your baseline, but also how you've moved away from it in different ways throughout the day. When the homeostatic balance in our nervous system shifts, we're not just more likely to have a raised baseline, we're also more likely to be easily affected by people, events, or circumstances, or indeed even the *anticipation* of any of these.

What's Triggering You?

The things that lead to these sudden increases in the activation of our nervous system are called triggers. For example, have you ever noticed that your nervous system can react to something before you've even had a conscious thought about it? Perhaps you meet someone for the first time and immediately dislike and feel unsafe with them. Or you're walking down the street minding your own business when you have a sudden sense that you need to speed up and get away from a certain person.

What's particularly interesting about the way we respond to these triggers is that it often happens outside of our conscious awareness. It isn't that we necessarily recognize something that happens and decide it's a threat to us. Instead, our unconscious is scanning the environment and deciding if we're safe or not, long before we can have any kind of conscious reflection about it. This is what Professor Porges calls neuroception.

However, what do you think informs the way your unconscious determines the cues from your environment? You've guessed it – the learned experiences from your own trauma history. The more unprocessed emotional trauma we have, the more likely it is that this is coloring and influencing how we're responding to the world around us. Indeed, the research clearly demonstrates that when we're in a fight, flight, or freeze state, we're more likely to misread the cues in our environment and, for example, to perceive someone with a neutral expression as being a danger to us.

Ultimately, there's a powerful confirmation bias in our unconscious in that it will actively look for and find danger signals where there are none as a way of attempting to keep us safe. This is one of the reasons why healing our trauma is so important – it allows us to learn to respond to the environment around us in a healthy and appropriate way once more.

The Nervous System Rating Scale

So, to recap, in the RESET model, your first step is to *recognize* which state your nervous system is in. Now that we've spent some time looking at the key ingredients of your nervous system, I want you to see this in the lived experience of your own body.

We want to understand more about how your nervous system evolves throughout the average day – i.e., what your baseline is, what your triggers are, and how they affect your baseline. Note that we're talking about normal day-to-day life here, not the exceptional circumstances when triggering a reaction in our nervous system might actually be necessary and appropriate.

As we explore this, it's very important to remember that each person's presentation of a maladaptive stress response is unique to them. However, there are some general patterns and trends that can help inform our understanding, and some people find using the scale below to rate their experience of their nervous system a helpful starting point.

Immobilization – Freeze

10. Completely numb and shut down

9. Disconnected and feelings hard to access

8. Demotivated and feeling stuck

Mobilization – Fight or Flight

7. Intense anxiety moving into feeling of resignation

6. Mind and body pumping with adrenaline and feeling wired

5. Mind racing, body feeling tense, and trying to think one's way to a feeling of safety

4. Feeling agitated and finding it hard to completely relax

Socialization – Healing State

3. Neutral feeling, but able to relax and enjoy the moment

2. Calm and relaxed and enjoying the company of others

1. Deep sense of relaxation and feeling safe within oneself

As you reflect on this nervous system rating scale, if you can see an easier or more accurate way to rate your own experience of your system, I'd encourage you to use it. This is about helping you to understand your own lived experience, not trying to manipulate it to fit that of some others I've just described.

Rate Your Nervous System Day-to-Day

Once you feel reasonably comfortable with the rating scale above, I'd like you to use it to rate your nervous system at certain times each day. I suggest doing this assessment for at least the next three days, but you can do it for longer if you find it helpful to have the additional information. You can download a worksheet to help with this in your companion course at www.alexhoward.com/trauma.

On waking: 1–10

Start of active day: 1–10

Lunchtime: 1–10

Mid-afternoon: 1–10

Early evening: 1–10

Bedtime: 1–10

During the night (if you wake): 1–10

Please note that there are no right or wrong scores here. This isn't about shaming yourself for where your nervous system is right now – it's about bringing more awareness so we can work on changing what's happening.

What did you discover from doing this assessment? Did you notice that your nervous system baseline was raised throughout the day, or perhaps there were particular times when there was an obvious increase in activation. Were you mostly in mobilization or immobilization, or did you have a healthy dose of being in a socialization/healing state?

For example, perhaps you noticed that you were activated around seeing a particular family member or doing a certain activity, or that as you became more tired later in the day, your resilience was lower. Ultimately, different things trigger different people.

The 'Anxiety Podcast'

The good news is that wherever your nervous system is right now, we can work together to reset it to a more normal level of functioning. Growing your awareness of what's currently happening is a key step toward this.

In my experience, when people complete the exercise that you've just done, they commonly say that they don't even know what's driving or triggering their nervous system – they just feel like they're in a perpetual, and at times all-consuming, state of anxiety. It's almost as if regardless of the content they're thinking about, the way they're thinking about it is from a perspective of anxiety.

It's a little like being tuned in to a podcast in which the guests might change but the core subject is always the same: anxiety. When we're tuned in to the 'anxiety podcast,' anxiety in its many and varied forms is what we get! If this is your experience, and there's just a constant sense of anxiety – sometimes in the background and sometimes in the foreground – please don't worry, because this is also part of what we're going to work on changing.

Are You in a Stress State or a Healing State?

When we're feeling overwhelmed and overstimulated in our nervous system, sometimes the last thing we need is a complex process of awareness and a practice to create change. If you're feeling like this right now, or in the future as you're working with this, the good news is that we can distil all of this down to one very simple question: In this moment, are you in a stress state or a healing state? Put another way: Are you in a mobilization or immobilization stress state or are you in a socialization/healing state?

Remember, for our body to heal, it has to be in a healing state. Whether it's our physical body or our emotional body, when it's in a stress state, our resources are directed to the demands of sustaining this state to keep us safe. This means those resources are not available for our healthy functioning in day-to-day life, let alone processing our trauma history and doing our healing work.

When we're in a healing state, our immense capacity for self-healing is unlocked. The more we work to retrain our homeostatic balance back to a healing state, the more we unlock this capacity. In our next step toward this, we're going to examine some of the personality patterns that are driving your nervous system away from a healing state.

CHAPTER 8

Examine Your Personality Patterns

When Monica first sat down in my clinic room, she did so with a weariness and heaviness that spoke volumes. I knew from her intake questionnaire that intense anxiety and a deep state of depression were what had brought her to see me, but clearly there was a lot more going on, too.

It soon became apparent that the despondency that emanated from Monica wasn't because she lacked the will to make changes in her life; instead, it was because that will had been pushed so hard and to little avail. Like many of us do, she'd tried everything she knew to improve her situation, but nothing had worked. With each effort to change, she felt a further reduction of the joy that had once filled her world.

As we explored Monica's life a little, I asked her what she did for work. She told me she was 'just a stay-at-home mum.' I gently interrupted her to ask, 'Just a stay-at-home mum?' She regarded me with a slightly dismissive expression, and then replied, 'Well, I used to be a lawyer in a top law firm, but my husband has a big job and with the three kids, one of us needed to be at home.'

I looked at Monica and said softly, 'You know, I also have three kids, and I come to work for a rest on Monday mornings after two days of parenting!' Her face softened a little as she continued to share the details of her daily life, and it became clear to me that Monica not only held impossible standards for herself, but she also seemed to place everyone else's needs above her own.

Trauma Outcomes in Action

Ultimately, Monica had learned that to be worthy of love, she had to become a perfect, virtually impossible-to-achieve version of herself, and becoming that wasn't only exhausting, it was also causing unsustainable pressure on her nervous system.

We talked about the history behind her need to be this idealized version of herself. She shared that her mother had been a successful doctor, and her father a decorated academic. She knew that her parents loved her, and they gave her many opportunities as a child. However, Monica also received a very clear message from her parents: The love you receive is in direct proportion to what you achieve, and if you don't feel loved, it's your fault.

If Monica scored 99 out of 100 in a test at school, her parents were more interested in the one question she'd got wrong than the 99 she'd answered correctly. If she came second in the class, what mattered was how she could be top next time, not the fact that she'd outperformed dozens of other children.

Furthermore, Monica had noticed that when she placed her parents' needs above her own, they would praise her heavily, and she'd feel closer and more connected to them. She shared a particular memory of this behavior from when she was around 10 years old. She'd come home from school upset about an incident with a friend and desperately needed comfort and time with one of her parents. However, they'd both been preoccupied with work, and so she'd hidden her feelings and played by herself. At bedtime, both parents praised her for being a 'big girl.'

When it came to Monica's relationship with her husband, it was the most natural thing in the world for her to consider his needs as more important than her own – from the big decisions like giving up her career to be with the children, to day-to-day things such as making sure he got to sleep in at the weekend. And Monica was desperate to give her children the unconditionally loving and accepting environment that she hadn't experienced, regardless of how overloaded or exhausted she might feel. From giving each child quality one-on-one time before bedtime, to cooking different meals to accommodate their food preferences, no act of service was too much.

But deep down, Monica often felt like a slave in her own home. She was overworked, underappreciated, and there was no end in sight. The more we dug into Monica's life, the more obvious it became to me that her anxiety wasn't a sign that something was broken, it was her nervous system functioning healthily to give her warning signs that her lifestyle was unsustainable.

A Love Deficit

Now, the details of your life may be very different to Monica's, but I'm guessing that some of her patterns might be familiar to you. Furthermore, what Monica had learned to do is something we all do in our own way.

You see, Monica had designed her life around the strategies she'd learned as a child to meet her three core emotional needs of boundaries, safety, and love. As we discussed earlier, as young children we're completely dependent on our primary caregivers to meet these needs for us, and as we get older, in time we must find other ways to meet them ourselves.

If our development as children was healthy, we'll have internalized positive messages from our caregivers. We will also have learned how to meet the three core emotional needs inside of ourselves, and so will not believe that they are dependent upon external events needing to happen or not happen. However, most of us have to develop various other strategies to find ways of meetings these needs, and these strategies themselves are often the source of enormous suffering in our lives.

In Monica's case, the primary emotional need she'd designed her life around meeting was love. And her learning was that to experience love, she had to elevate everyone else's needs above her own – she had to become a 'helper.' She'd also learned that the more she achieved, be it in her career as a lawyer or by trying to be a 'supermom,' the more love she'd receive.

Monica's depression and anxiety were due in part to the huge pressure she was placing on herself, but they were also down to the fact that however hard she worked, her core needs were not actually being met. The love deficit she felt was still driving her life.

The Idealized Self

Just like Monica, we all have stories and ideas about the person we need to be for the world to meet our core emotional needs. Perhaps we need to do things perfectly right, or perhaps we always need to be seen to be in control of what's happening. Or perhaps, like Monica, we need to make our life a masterpiece of achievements or be a helper with endless patience.

This person we need to become is our 'idealized self.' Sometimes this idealized self is a slight detour from our true self, and other times there's a giant chasm between the two which becomes a huge source of day-to-day suffering as we try to traverse it.

The really sad thing about our intense battle to become this idealized self is that it's a relatively fruitless one to fight. Even if we're temporarily successful in meeting our emotional needs in this way, in doing so, we're actually creating two rather major problems. The first is that we're still dependent on someone else or the environment around us to meet the need. The second is that the place we truly must have the need met is in our relationship with ourselves.

The Five Key Personality Patterns

Now of course there are as many different idealized selves as there are people on Earth because we're all unique in our own individual expressions. But at the same time, there are some common personality patterns with which it's helpful to become familiar to create more awareness around our own patterns. Let's spend some time exploring five of these now.

1: Helper

Let's start with one of Monica's key patterns, the helper. The helper pattern is where we regard other people's needs as more important than our own, and it becomes our responsibility to meet their needs for them. It can also be that we've learned that by meeting the needs of others, we'll then be safe – this is known as 'fawning.'

For example, imagine that you're travelling home from work after a particularly long day and you're feeling in desperate need of some quality downtime before you call it an early night. A mindless TV show alongside a healthy takeout is just what the doctor ordered.

Halfway through your journey, you receive a text message from a friend asking if you'll go over to their place for the evening. They've had a crappy day, they explain, and want some company. Now, it's obvious that your friend isn't in some sort of immediate and intense distress that may justify changing your plans. In fact, they're in a similar space to you, except they want company, and you want time alone.

Governed by your helper pattern, though, you don't give this a second thought, and you redirect your journey to be there for them. After all, their needs are more important than your own, and this is the pattern around which your life's been designed. The result may well be that your friend feels better, but at what cost to you?

The helper pattern can play out in micro ways such as this, but also in macro ways, including in the career we choose, or how our intimate relationship is set up. And if you recall that being in a maladaptive stress response can distort how we read the cues in the environment around us, what often also happens with the helper pattern is that we interpret others' struggles as a need for our input, when they might be just fine as they are. And in fact, what we're often doing is teaching others to become dependent on us.

Here are some common beliefs held by someone with the helper pattern.

- **Boundaries:** If I look after those around me, they'll look after me and respect my boundaries and needs.

- **Safety:** If I make myself indispensable to others, they won't threaten me or my sense of safety.

- **Love:** If I meet your needs, you'll love me.

2: Achiever

The other pattern we explored with Monica's story is that of the achiever. Achievers believe that their sense of value as a person is tied to what they do and achieve in the world. Often, they've had childhood experiences of feeling that healthy boundaries, safety, and love were connected to their achievements, and their life can become a constant, relentless pursuit of achievement in a painful bid to meet the need.

The stereotypical example of an achiever is someone who's driven by their career and financial status, but this is just one of many. Achiever patterns can play out in anything from being the best parent to being the most impactful eco-activist. For some people, the achiever pattern can also manifest in being an anti-achiever, and effectively celebrating not being defined by external things. However, in a sense, it's the same pattern, just in rejection of achievement.

The key principle with the achiever pattern is that we believe there are things we can make happen on the outside that will change how we feel on the inside. And the more we make those things happen, the more we can meet our core emotional needs.

Here are some common beliefs held by those with an achiever pattern.

- **Boundaries**: If I'm successful, I can do what I want.

- **Safety**: The more successful I am, the less dependent I'll be on others.

- **Love**: The more I achieve, the more others will love me.

3: Perfectionist

The perfectionist pattern is a close relative of the achiever pattern. Perfectionists put a disproportionate focus on getting things right; whereas the achiever is driven by reaching the destination, perfectionists are motivated to get the details right along the way.

The perfectionist pattern will have us obsessing over small details, inflating them to a disproportionate sense of importance. This can play out in everything from our performance at work to our personal appearance, or in the way we communicate with others. Examples might be obsessing over our body image, or a relentless focus on spelling and grammar in writing, in a way that actually obstructs our progress.

When we have a perfectionist pattern, we often also have an acute sense of right and wrong. We can be particularly judgmental and harsh in our thoughts and actions toward those we believe are wrong, and we can feel an inflated sense of superiority. This can sometimes create more distance from those around us than, deep in our heart, we'd like.

Here are some common beliefs we may have with a perfectionist pattern.

- **Boundaries**: Being right gives me the legitimacy to set and hold my boundaries.

- **Safety**: If I do things perfectly, I won't be vulnerable to criticism.

- **Love**: I need to be perfect to be lovable.

4: Controller

The controller pattern is about being seen as strong and in control. This can play out in needing to be in control of the people and circumstances in the environment around us, but also of our own internal state.

In a healthier expression this pattern can present as being highly capable as a leader; however, a less healthy version will see people being manipulated or bullied to suit the needs of the controller. Because of the need to control their internal state, controllers also find it very hard to show any kind of emotion or vulnerability.

One of the things that's so stressful about living with a controller pattern is that ultimately, we cannot control the world around us. The constant attempts to do so, and the endless efforts to predict our environment, become incredibly depleting and are a fruitless task.

Here are some common beliefs we may have with a controller pattern.

- **Boundaries**: If I'm in control, no one will be able to threaten my boundaries.

- **Safety**: The way to be safe is to be in control.

- **Love**: If I protect and stand up for others, I'll be lovable.

5: Peacekeeper

The peacekeeper pattern is in many ways the opposite of the controller pattern. With this pattern, we'll choose peace and harmony over directness and confrontation. This will often involve ignoring and rejecting our own needs for the convenience and comfort of those around us. Conflict and disagreement are our Kryptonite, and we'll work as hard as we can to create circumstances that won't make people feel uncomfortable.

The cost, of course, is that the more we work to create harmony and ease for those around us, the more we must reject and ignore our own needs and emotions. Almost by definition, asking for and expressing our needs would risk offending someone or putting them out, and so it's easier for us to blend into the background and prioritize the needs of others in the group.

Here are some common beliefs we may hold in a peacekeeper pattern.

- **Boundaries**: By keeping the peace, I'll be in harmony with others.

- **Safety**: If I accommodate other people's needs, they'll protect me and keep me safe.

- **Love**: The easier I am to get along with, the more people will love me.

Please note that this isn't an exhaustive list of personality patterns and there are many variations to how these patterns might show up in our lives; and of course, they can do so to varying degrees. It's also important to bear in mind that you'll likely have several, or perhaps even all, of these patterns. That's just fine. What's key is that the more aware of them you become, the more empowered you'll be to do something different.

Who's Your Idealized Self?

In this exercise, the goal is to understand as best you can the person you believe you need to be to get your core emotional needs met. Please remember, this isn't about self-judgement or criticism – it's about bringing fresh awareness to help empower you to change. Answer the following questions as honestly as you can using the worksheet at www.alexhoward.com/trauma.

- For you and others to respect your boundaries, who do you believe you need to be?
- To feel safe in the world, who do you believe you need to be?
- To feel loved and adored by others, who do you believe you need to be?

As you answer these questions, please bear in mind the five personality patterns we explored above. Do you need to help, achieve, perfect, control, or peace-keep to feel boundaried, safe, and loved in the world? You can find a full checklist of the personality patterns in your companion course at www.alexhoward.com/trauma.

Taking Back Our Power

I often find when working with people that when they can make sense of *why* they feel the way they do, it's a key step in taking back some of the power. Returning to Monica one last time, as she came to realize that at the heart of her compulsive helper and achiever patterns was a deep need to feel safe and loved, something started to soften. For the first time in years, she didn't feel as if she was going crazy; instead, she recognized that the way she was approaching her life was causing an untenable level of stress that was consistently pushing her nervous system into overdrive.

However, it was also obvious that this awareness alone wasn't enough to retrain a nervous system that had been programmed over decades. Indeed, it was where we're going next in our journey that was so important for creating lasting change for Monica and ultimately transformed her life.

CHAPTER 9
Stop Running, Start Feeling

There's a well-known joke in therapy circles: How many therapists does it take to change a light bulb? Only one, but the light bulb must *want* to change. Put another way, if a patient doesn't change, it's their fault because they aren't sufficiently motivated to do so. No one lays responsibility at the door of the therapist or considers whether their therapeutic methodology is the right one for the patient, and to me, this is a cop-out at best, and victim blaming at worst.

Sanaya was in her early twenties when she agreed to become part of my *In Therapy with Alex Howard* YouTube series. Considering that at the time she was crippled by feelings of anxiety and occasionally experienced intense panic attacks, I particularly admired her for being willing to allow her therapeutic journey with me to be filmed.

To ensure that they are robust enough to go through the process, and that their motivations are aligned with those of the series, all participants have an independent psychological assessment before we start filming. The psychologist's report for Sanaya had stated that she hadn't connected with her previous therapists, who had questioned her motivation and goals for therapy. Was she really committed to changing? In their eyes, Sanaya was the aforementioned light bulb.

What I observed in our first session, however, wasn't a young woman who didn't *want* to change, but one who was afraid of what might be involved in changing, and whether it would even be possible. Sanaya was also deeply afraid of *not* changing and continuing in the anxiety hell in which she was trapped.

An Inner State of Safety

In my experience with clients, for any therapeutic work to be effective – let alone for them to feel able to open to their hidden and unprocessed emotions – they must first feel safe. They need to feel safe with the therapist, safe with the method, and as part of the therapeutic work, learn how to create a feeling of safety in themselves that isn't dependent on others. Effectively, they need to move from co-regulation with the therapist to self-regulation for themselves.

Returning to our proverbial light bulb, perhaps it only takes one therapist to help it change, but they need to help it feel safe enough to do so. After all, safety isn't just a nice thing to have, it's the very foundation of what we need to heal.

Sanaya's ongoing state of anxiety meant that when she looked at herself, her feelings, and the world around her, everything was perceived through the lens of fear. The 'anxiety podcast' was playing in every situation in which she found herself. The prospect of changing was terrifying, but so was not changing. And even if she could change, would it last? And would she even like the person she became? Trapped between a rock and a hard place, everywhere she looked there was a trigger to her nervous system.

And of course, Sanaya wasn't alone in her experience. This is a dilemma that many of us experience along the way – to feel safe enough to change we need to be able to calm our nervous system, but to calm our nervous system we need to change. And so, when it comes to truly learning to feel and connect to our emotions, we first need to learn to create an inner state of safety.

Self-Regulating Our Nervous System

Having an inner state of safety is a superpower that will not only transform your trauma healing, but it will also revolutionize your relationship with the world around you. So, where does the inner feeling of safety we need come from and how do we create it?

As we touched on in Chapter 4, an inner state of safety is created when we're able to self-regulate our nervous system in response to the world. In the context of our nervous system, self-regulation means that we have direct influence over our physiological and emotional state. It doesn't mean we can control how we feel in any given moment, but it does mean that if we recognize that our nervous system is running too fast, we have the capacity to actively slow it down and come to a calmer place.

In an ideal world, we're given this as a gift from our primary caregivers (most commonly our mother) as a baby[1-3] and as we grow.[4,5] As we find ourselves impacted and affected by the world around us, our caregivers soothe us, not just in their words and actions but, most importantly, by their own calm and settled nervous system.

By co-regulating with our caregivers, we learn that the world is a safe place, and crucially, we learn how to do the same for ourselves and self-regulate our system to create an inner state of safety. Just as we're learning to walk, talk, and do a million other incredible things, our nervous system is also learning how to self-regulate in response to our environment.

However, to varying degrees, many of us didn't have this need met in the way we needed to.[6-11] Indeed, as we discussed earlier, this shift in our homeostatic balance is one of the ECHOs of trauma. And so, when it comes to resetting our nervous system, the skill of self-regulation is the foundation. Thankfully, like all skills, with practice, we can learn to do it. Let's look at that now.

Anxiety About Anxiety

Tracking back to Sanaya's story, one of her most challenging triggers was noticing the feeling of anxiety in her body and this then triggering more anxiety. In a sense, her maladaptive stress response was self-generating. The more anxiety she felt, the more anxious she'd become. This is what I call anxiety about anxiety.

When our maladaptive stress response results in an excess of stress hormones, such as cortisol and adrenaline, being released, it'll take some time for our blood chemistry to normalize. When I explained this process to Sanaya, it helped her to understand that measuring any intervention by whether she felt different immediately wasn't realistic. Instead, she needed to learn to find a place of acceptance in the short term, and to then notice things settling in her body a few minutes later. You'll find a video of this exchange with Sanaya in your free companion course at www.alexhoward.com/trauma.

When it comes to learning to self-regulate our nervous system, the most calming thing we can experience is discovering that we can directly impact our own state. The more influence we realize we have, the less powerless we feel, and the calmer our system will become.

How Meditation Can Help

Dozens if not hundreds of different tools have been developed over the years to help us learn to self-regulate our nervous system, and almost all of them have their roots in mindfulness and meditation practice. In fact, one of the most researched psychological tools in the history of science is the practice of meditation.[12–16] Over the last few decades, awareness around meditation has grown hugely, and so much of that is positive.

It's also worth noting that not all forms of meditation have the same benefits and focuses. For example, practices such as Transcendental Meditation are designed to help us cultivate a trance-like state of bliss, and visualization practices may focus on impacting certain feeling states. Although these are both helpful, they are not necessarily the quickest path to cultivating a feeling of inner safety.

Training a New Way of Being

In the form of meditation that we're about to explore the key thing is to shift your focus from your mind into being present with your body. Ultimately, you're working to become more deeply connected to your immediate experience, without trying to disconnect or change it. Learning to relax into your body helps you to move from thinking to feeling. Remember, you can't *think* your way to a *feeling* of safety. But you can *feel* your way to a *feeling* of safety.

As the writer James Redfield so potently put it, 'Where attention goes, energy flows.' By training your attention into your body, gradually you're training your energy out of your mind and over-activated nervous system and into the place where the feeling of safety we ultimately crave exists. By learning to stop running and start feeling, we can come home to our body and make peace with whatever we're experiencing.

Ultimately, self-regulation isn't about attempting to change or fix what's happening; instead, it's about coming to a place of acceptance and peace with it. By moving our attention from feeding the problem to actively calming our system in the moment, we're training a new way of being.

Now, part of the challenge is that you likely have decades of conditioning that's trained your mind to be a certain way. As we'll discuss in the next chapter, it's going to take time to train it into a different way of functioning. Not because you're doing the practice wrongly, but because your brain is attempting to return to what it believes is balance.

Remember also that when we're in a maladaptive stress response a natural speeding-up occurs to engage our nervous system and disconnect us from our emotions. And so, by learning to meditate we're again working against a deeply ingrained instinct.

Keeping It Simple

When it comes to meditation, my preference is to keep the practice as simple as possible. In fact, the participants on my RESET Program® consistently report that because of the straightforward, structured method at the heart of the way I teach meditation, they've been able to sustain a consistent practice for the first time.

Some meditation practices are centuries old, so it's not surprising that there are often steps and elements to them that exist because of the history, not because they're designed to make meditation accessible. With some schools of meditation, it can take decades to reach a level of mastery in certain intricate elements. Some of these aspects are important refinements for experienced meditators, and others are just the way they are because that's how they were passed down.

For example, some schools of meditation insist on the practice of certain postures, including cross-legged ones. These might lend themselves well to people living in warm climates and with highly active lifestyles, but they don't always work for those in cold, damp Western countries where many people have sedentary jobs, or for those with mobility issues. Indeed, I'm aware of several people who have sustained quite unpleasant injuries while trying repeatedly to force themselves into these postures when clearly their body wasn't a willing participant.

Mastering the Basics

Over the years, my approach to teaching meditation has been to find the 'minimum effective dose' – asking, what's the lowest number of key principles we can strip the practice back to, while allowing us to have the maximum impact? I also think it's important to design our meditation training in a way which sets us up for success. Calming the mind and connecting to the body might sound straightforward, but it can sometimes be the hardest thing in the world to do, and the more nuances we must struggle with to get it right, the more overwhelming it becomes.

If we begin by mastering the basics, over time we can add in more elements to help take our practice to the next level. Conversely, if we start by overloading ourselves with details, we may never get the basics right, and soon give up in frustration. Sometimes, trying to do everything perfectly correctly can be a sign that the perfectionist pattern we explored in the last chapter is playing out.

I'm also aware that you may follow a prayer or meditation practice linked to a religious path. It's important to say that what we're going to practice together is respectful of all paths but linked to none. What we'll be focusing on are the scientific elements of meditation that have been demonstrated time and again to play a key role in helping us to self-regulate our nervous system.

Trauma-Informed Meditation

Many people working on healing their trauma find that meditation is a hugely helpful practice for learning to calm and ground their mind, emotions, and body. However, for some it can be particularly difficult, and taking a different approach can be beneficial.

When trauma has led to a dysregulated mind and nervous system, and we come into close contact with this through meditation, we can become increasingly frustrated and triggered by how quickly everything's running. Sitting still and observing our mind and body effectively sends us in a loop of running too fast, feeling frustrated about running too fast, and then running faster in response.

In this instance, moving meditation can be immensely helpful. In a sense, allowing the energy in our system to move, or indeed moving with it, makes it easier for the system to become calm and to reset. There are many forms of moving meditation, including walking meditation, yoga, Tai Chi, and Qigong.[17] Sometimes, starting with a practice such as these before then moving into a sitting meditation can make all the difference.

We may also have trauma triggers relating to our emotional or physical body that can become overwhelming or even retraumatizing during standard mind/body practices.[18-20] In these cases it's important to use approaches that help us to maintain a sense of being grounded and connected to what feels safe, while exploring our inner world and sensations.[21]

Emotional processing approaches such as Emotional Freedom Technique (EFT/Tapping), and Eye Movement Desensitization and Reprocessing (EMDR) can also be very helpful with the guidance of an experienced and trauma-informed practitioner.[22-24]

It's also worth noting that although closing our eyes during meditation will often help our practice, as we'll have less visual sensory input to distract us and draw our attention, for some people doing so will be triggering. If this is true for you, it's fine to keep your eyes open, but do pick a spot on the wall on which to hold a soft gaze, as this will help prevent your eyes being drawn to distractions.

The Key Principles of Meditation

Basically, there are four key intentions we're trying to achieve through meditation, and three tactics we'll be deploying to help us do so. Let's explore each of these in turn.

Four Intentions

1. **Turn attention inward:** In much of our day-to-day life, our attention is almost entirely on the world around us and what's happening in it. We may have all kinds of thoughts and responses during this, but our primary focus is on what's happening outside us. With meditation we're aiming to shift our attention away from external events and toward our internal experience.

2. **Move attention from mind to body:** Most of us experience ourselves from the neck upward. We're so caught up in our thoughts and mental responses to the world around us that the lived experience of our body is mostly outside our conscious awareness. Through our meditation practice, we're working to retrain our attention away from being so fixated on our mind, to being more connected to the felt sense of our body.

3. **Slow system down:** For many of us, part of the problem is that our mind and nervous system are running too quickly. When we're learning to meditate, we want to slow down our system and to feel the sense of presence and holding that comes from being connected to the present moment. And, as we'll discuss in the coming chapters, when our system's running at a healthier speed, it's also much easier to connect to and process our emotions.

4. **Hold attention steady:** The maladaptive stress response will have our mind in lots of places at once, and easily triggered by the smallest thing. Remember the definition of homeostasis: 'same' and 'stable.' By holding our attention steady, we're helping to retrain our own internal world to have more elements of this homeostatic balance. By learning

to stay with our experience, and not being so easily triggered by events and circumstances, we're bringing ourselves back to this place of inner safety.

You don't have to think about these key principles while you're meditating, but I believe that having an understanding of our orientation is both helpful and important. Let's now explore the three tactics we're going to deploy in our meditation practice.

Three Tactics

1. **Observe breath.** By learning to observe the quality of our breath during meditation – such as its speed and the sensation of air filling our lungs – we're giving our attention somewhere to go, while also growing our focus on our body. Our breath is also something that's happening in the present moment, which is another important part of bringing our attention into what's true now, and out of our hooks into the traumas of the past.

2. **Let go of thoughts.** As we touched on above with anxiety about anxiety, thoughts can very easily become self-generating. One thought will lead to another and another and before we know it, we're on a completely different track of thought from where we started. However, we're not in control of where our thinking is going. The goal of meditation isn't to try and stop specific thoughts, but to move our focus and attention away from them and onto the object of our meditation (in this instance, our breath). In a sense we're allowing our thoughts to be there, but we're not making them the primary focus of our current experience.

3. **Sense body.** By putting our mind on the immediate sensations in our body, once again we're able to focus on something that's happening in this moment, in real time. We're also supporting the movement

of our attention away from what's happening in our mind and into the felt experience of our body. Remember, where attention goes, energy flows.

How to Meditate

Let's now start to play with meditation itself. You can do the following practice with your eyes open or closed. It's often helpful to do it sitting up with a straight spine and your feet on the floor. If you're more comfortable lying down that's also fine, but be mindful that if you fall asleep, that isn't the same as meditation practice – although, of course, it's hugely valuable in itself!

Your Basic Meditation Practice

If you're new to meditation, I'd recommend starting off with just five minutes of practice. If you have some experience, you can of course spend more time on it. Remember that we want to set you up for success, so this is about cultivating positive experiences on which to build, not trying to set meditation records!

1. Take some time to focus your attention on your breath. Notice the quality of your inhale and exhale and trace the feeling of the air through your body.

2. As you do this, notice your thoughts and the focuses of your mind. As you become aware of the tracks of thought your mind is on, bring your attention back to your breath. You're not trying to stop your thoughts. Instead, you're choosing to direct your attention toward your breath.

3. If you find it helpful, count your breaths. You can count 1 for the inhale, 2 for the exhale, and so on. When you reach 10, start again. If you forget which number you're on, don't worry, just start counting again, from 1.

4. While you're maintaining your focus on your breath, slowly move your attention to feeling the sensations in your body. There's no right or wrong experience to be having here – your goal is ultimately to be present to what's there. You're not judging or trying to fix what you're experiencing; you're simply patiently observing it with your attention.

5. When you reach the end of your practice time, allow yourself to gently bring your attention back into the room and notice how you feel now.

This practice is incredibly simple, but like many simple things it's not always easy. Ultimately, it's much easier to learn to meditate by being guided through it, so, as part of your free companion course (www.alexhoward. com/trauma), I've recorded some guided meditations to support you, using this approach.

Practice Leads to Lasting Change

Whatever you experience when you first start to meditate is fine – there are no right or wrong experiences. Perhaps you felt that nothing shifted in your nervous system through doing this practice. If that's the case, please don't worry, just keep going. It may also be that you felt more activated in your system. If so, remember what I said earlier about moving meditation, along with the importance of doing some trauma healing beforehand.

Even in the best-case scenario, where you may notice a shift in your nervous system and feel a little calmer immediately after practicing, you'll likely find that as soon as you stop, your nervous system will gradually reactivate back to its stress state. Remember, this is because it believes that's normal – it's the homeostatic balance it's normalized to. To create lasting change, you must be diligent, consistent, and patient with your meditation practice over time. Once you're consistently practicing for five minutes, you can start to build, ideally up to at least 30 minutes a day.

Ultimately, meditation practice is so called because practice is exactly what's needed to create lasting change. Over time, as you keep bringing your nervous system back to a state of calmness and connection to your body, you're teaching your system that this is the new homeostatic balance, and the place from which you now want to live.

Being with Discomfort

One of the challenges of connecting to our body and emotions is that we might start to feel some of the feelings that our maladaptive stress response has been helping us escape from. We'll drill into this in much more detail in the coming few chapters, but for now please know that this isn't a sign that something's wrong; in fact, it's often a sign of the progress you've been working so hard to achieve.

Part of the art of learning to self-regulate our nervous system is allowing our experience to be as it is. Just as a soothing and loving parent reassures a small child, we're sending the message to our own physical and emotional bodies that our experience is OK, and so are we.

Whether or not we feel that we're mastering the simple but not easy practice of meditation, this learning to be with and meet our feelings and emotions from a calm and welcoming place can itself be transformational. Indeed, it's the comfort and holding that our emotional body needs for it to trust us enough to open to us. And, by learning to give this gift to ourselves, we're truly becoming a healthy and balanced adult in the world.

Breaking the Cycle

Let's return to Sanaya's story one last time. Alongside some other elements, which you're learning in this book, meditation played a hugely helpful role in calming her anxiety. Breaking the cycle of anxiety triggering more anxiety and learning how to self-regulate her nervous system meant that she was no longer at the mercy of her panic attacks, and she could start to bring her true personality and talents to the world.

By the end of our eight filmed sessions together, Sanaya was full of joy and excitement for her future and had landed her dream internship in the film industry. As I said to her in our last session, the key wasn't that she'd never feel anxiety again, but that she now had the tools to self-regulate her nervous system in response to it, which is the ultimate freedom in life.

CHAPTER 10

Put a STOP to Your Unhelpful Behaviors

According to surveys, three-quarters of us have a fear of public speaking; in fact, in some, it's ranked higher than the fear of death. In the early part of my career, I found myself in the rather fortunate group of people who enjoyed speaking in public. At the age of 23, I travelled around the UK promoting my first book, sometimes speaking to a handful of people, other times to hundreds. I loved the buzz it gave me, and the opportunity to connect with readers.

Utilizing the skills I'd learned along the way, a few years later I had an unexpected side gig as a corporate speaker, offering a message of personal resilience and commitment. From time to time, I'd be brought in to speak at corporate training events, and I enjoyed the variety it brought to my day-to-day life as a therapist.

However, at the height of the period in my life when I was suffering from intense anxiety and panic attacks, which I described in the first chapter, I was booked to speak to around 100 salespeople at an event aboard the old battleship HMS *Belfast* on London's River Thames.

In the preceding few months my anxiety had become so crippling that leaving the house was challenging enough, let alone being on display in a room full of people. The obvious solution would have been to cancel the event; however, a rather toxic marriage between my achiever and helper patterns meant I didn't want to be seen as weak, or to be letting anyone down.

Perhaps as life's way of trying to protect me from what was coming, I got stuck in traffic while driving across London to the event. When I finally arrived, there were just a few minutes remaining until I was due to speak, and my already severe anxiety had gone into overdrive. Hoping that the intense cortisol and adrenaline rush would see me through, I took to the stage feeling as if all I wanted to do was run from the building.

Learning an Unhelpful Behavioral Pattern

It's not unusual to feel nervous at the start of a presentation. It often takes both speaker and audience a few minutes to relax and settle into each other, and to find a natural groove. The problem was, on this occasion, the settling in wasn't coming for me. In fact, the opposite was happening.

I could feel that my voice wasn't loose; I found it impossible to focus on the audience; and working the stage became a rather frantic pacing as I tried to move the energy of the intense panic that was growing in me. To say I was in extreme fight or flight was an understatement, but worse than that, I was about to go into shutdown.

When I noticed that my voice had started to shake, things unraveled. I realized that the confident act I was so desperately trying to present was starting to crack. And when you're talking about resilience, drive, and motivation while at the same time having a panic attack, the message you're selling becomes somewhat empty. As fight or flight turned to freeze, I was unable to draw breath or get my voice out.

At this point conscious control was gone, and instinct took over. I walked off the stage, and what happened next was interesting. I sat on a chair and managed to take a few deep breaths. As much as I wanted to run to my car and drive home, something else kicked in. Somehow, I knew that if I didn't go back out and finish my presentation it might be the last time that I ever spoke in public. Despite the hell I was living through, that was a price I wasn't willing to pay.

Driven by sheer willpower, I picked up my chair and put it in the middle of the stage, fearing that I might pass out if I stood. I then carried on with my presentation. A few minutes later I did finally start to settle a bit, completely blocking out in my mind what had just happened. I was back on my feet, and I knew I could get through the remainder of the hour. I managed to finish the presentation, and I received a standing ovation. So, on some level, I'd pulled it off.

Unfortunately, in the years that followed, the ECHOs of that experience were dramatic. I found myself joining the 75 percent of the population who fear public speaking, and although I had to continue doing so for parts of my work, I actively avoided saying yes to anything that wasn't essential for several years.

The problem was that my nervous system had learned a new pattern. It had coded public speaking as dangerous, and that meant that my stress levels were off the chart at the very thought of it. And of course, the more this happened, the more the pattern was reinforced.

How the Brain Creates Our Habits and Behavior

One of the miracles of being human is our ability to make sense of and orient ourselves in an increasingly complex and fast-moving world. In Chapter 6 we talked about our beliefs and how we develop simplifications of the world around us to help us navigate our journey through it. Well, our unconscious learns to repeat these patterns which it believes will keep us safe.

On a neurological level, these beliefs are effectively habits in our thinking that become wired into our brain. Our neurons (brain cells) literally build connections to help certain thinking patterns run more effectively. Like constructing a highway to bypass a city, our brain builds neurological connections to speed up its effectiveness.

In 1949, Canadian neuroscientist Donald Hebb coined the phrase 'neurons that fire together, wire together.' By this he meant that the more we use a certain neural circuit, the stronger than circuit becomes. It's through this process that we embed certain ways of thinking, which is why just *wanting* something to be different is often not enough to change it. Put simply, our brain is shaped by the patterns we run, and this process is referred to as neuro (brain) plasticity (shaped).

In the case of my experience of public speaking, in the years following the initial event, my brain continued to code public speaking as dangerous, and so I built a super-fast pathway to trigger a stress response, even if I just anticipated having to speak. And it became a self-fulfilling prophecy – the more it happened, the stronger the pathway became.

Why Compassion Matters

Being aware of the way our brain creates habits and behaviors and wires itself to reinforce them is important not just for understanding how to initiate change, but also for bringing more compassion to the situation. When it comes to addictions, for example, beyond the often-emotional needs and drivers fueling them, there's usually a very deeply ingrained habit in the brain and nervous system.

It's easy for someone who isn't addicted to nicotine, say, to sit in judgement of those who are struggling to stop smoking. But when someone's brain is wired to reach for cigarettes as a way to change their emotional state, and it's also a core program for functioning in their day-to-day life, stopping is that much more difficult. Indeed, there are likely numerous triggers in different situations, all of which lead to the same action – smoking. And when this choice is taken away, in the short term the whole system is thrown out of balance, which is likely yet another trigger to smoke.

Although of course a level of discipline and motivation is required for us to make changes, we also need to remember that one person's nicotine might be another person's need for exercise, and that it can take some time and skill to learn to interrupt and rewire our programming. The harsher we become with ourselves, the more likely we are to default to the pattern we're trying to change. So, finding a way to meet our unhelpful habits with kindness and empathy is often an important part of the change.

Retraining Our Nervous System

The good news is that the science of neuroplasticity clearly demonstrates that our behavioral patterns can be rewired.[1,2] Although it can take some diligence, patience, and skill to train a new pattern, if we work to condition ourselves toward a new way of functioning, in time this can become our default.

Furthermore, the research on brain cells is fascinating. Although it's true that as we age our neurons gradually atrophy, in fact, we have 10 times more brain capacity than was previously thought.[3] And what's most important is that we can create new neural pathways throughout our lives. Indeed, after Albert Einstein died, it was discovered that his parietal lobes (the top, back part of his brain) were 15 percent larger than average. Like a muscle, our brain responds to challenge.

When we actively work to change a behavioral pattern, initially it takes some effort and focus because we're working against programming that might have been running for decades. Furthermore, the new pattern will feel unfamiliar and even uncomfortable. But in time, we're building new neural pathways. To build these new pathways, we need to actively work to retrain our nervous system. Just as we do when developing a new skill, we go through a series of stages to install a new behavioral pattern. These are:

- **Unconscious incompetence** – we don't know what we don't know: i.e., we don't know that the pattern we want to change is a problem.

- **Conscious incompetence** – we know what we don't know, but we don't have other options available.

- **Conscious competence** – we have a new pattern available, but it takes conscious effort to do it.

- **Unconscious competence** – the new pattern requires almost no conscious effort and can run unconsciously.

How to STOP a Behavioral Pattern

At the stage of conscious competence, we're particularly vulnerable to giving up and feeling as if we don't have what it takes. But the key is to stay with the pattern to train our nervous system until it becomes the new, unconscious competence. In neuroplasticity terms, we need to wire in the new pathway.

Ultimately, what we need is a way to catch and interrupt our existing unhelpful behavioral patterns. In my online RESET Program® this is something we spend significant time on, bringing in specific techniques we've developed within the Therapeutic Coaching® methodology. However, a simple way to introduce some of the key elements is to learn to STOP the existing pattern and create a new way of being:

1. See the pattern

2. Take a pause

3. Open to your physical and emotional bodies

4. Praise yourself

Let's explore this four-step process.

1: See the Pattern

We've talked a lot already about the importance of awareness and learning to see the patterns we're running, particularly in Chapter 8, where we explored the five personality patterns. At this point you're likely sick of me saying 'If you can see it, you don't have to be it,' but the more general awareness we build of the pattern we're running, the greater the probability we can see it in real time as it happens. By seeing the pattern in real time, we're able to do something about it.

2: Take a Pause

Once we see the pattern we're running, we then need to take a pause and shift the state in our nervous system. When a pattern of thinking or behavior has momentum, particularly if our nervous system is triggered, the last thing we might feel like doing is pausing, but it's also the thing that's most likely to make the difference.

By switching into a different mode – i.e., moving back to a state of socialization, back into a healing state, we're breaking the pattern and teaching our nervous system a different response. Taking a pause can be as simple as taking a deep breath.

3: Open to Your Physical and Emotional Bodies

As you take a pause, the next thing is to open your attention to what's happening in your physical and emotional bodies. The first step is to ground yourself and connect to the moment. Remember, the sensations and experiences of our physical and emotional bodies are our gateway to the present moment.

The second thing this will do is allow you to start to work with whatever it is that you may have been disconnecting from and trying to escape from. By giving that which needs attention your *real* attention, things can start to open up and change. We'll explore this further in the next chapter.

4: Praise Yourself

As you do the previous step, you then want to praise yourself for the new direction you're going in. Apart from creating a softer and more supportive inner landscape, this gentle reinforcement helps to create a new pattern of talking to yourself in a different way.

Praising yourself can be as simple as saying *well done*, or *very good*, to yourself. Although you may be tempted to skip this step, please don't. Indeed, those of us who are the most likely not to give ourselves positive reinforcement are probably the ones who need it the most.

You can do this STOP process proactively – i.e., thinking about upcoming situations and then practicing in your mind responding differently – and you can do it reactively in the moment as you find yourself stuck in a particular thought pattern.

I know that the STOP process sounds very simple, but in many ways, it's this very simplicity which makes it so effective. When we're looking to change an existing pattern, if we need to go through a long and complex inner process each time, it won't have the necessary effect of teaching our nervous system to do something different.

By having a very clear message to change focus, we're actively rewiring our brain to go in a different direction, and training this as the new pattern. And remember, we're learning new habits and patterns all the time anyway – the difference here is that we're doing so deliberately and consciously. Ultimately, you're learning to train unconscious competence to wire the new pattern into your brain and nervous system.

Conditioning the Change

In terms of catching and interrupting an existing pattern, the speed at which we do so also matters. The longer we let the unhelpful pattern of thinking or behavior run, the stronger that neural pathway becomes. The faster and the more consistently we catch the pattern, interrupt it, and move to a new thought or behavior, the better we are at training this as the new pathway.

Consistently catching our patterns takes a certain amount of discipline and commitment to our healing work. And the more we invest in changing these patterns, the easier it will then be to do so, as we'll have some momentum with the new neural pathway.

In time, what you'll likely notice is that this process becomes a natural response for you. Whereas initially you had to work hard to even see the patterns, let alone shift your state, in time the process almost does it itself. Indeed, that's neuroplasticity in action!

Opening to Deeper Healing

Now, I'm mindful that as you read this you might be thinking, this is all well and good, but how about the deeper emotional healing that we might need as part of our trauma healing? Well, that's exactly where we're about to go. But please don't underestimate the importance of this work in preparation.

By learning to come back to our physical and emotional bodies more consistently, we're also training our nervous system to have a different homeostasis. In the same way that our nervous system has been unconsciously shaped by years of life experiences, the power of this work is that you can now learn to consciously train a different way of living and feeling in your nervous system. It takes practice and patience to do so, but the possible outcomes have the potential to be life changing.

This was certainly the case for Monica (who you met in Chapter 8) when it came to transforming her depression and anxiety. She found the STOP process particularly helpful. Multiple times throughout the day she'd catch herself rushing to the next activity or ignoring her own needs. As she did, she worked hard to change her default response.

For example, she would See the pattern of pushing beyond her limits and would Take a pause by stopping for a moment and having a few deep breaths. She'd then Open to her physical and emotional bodies by doing a mini-meditation and slowing everything down. Finally, she'd Praise herself by acknowledging the changes she was making.

The more Monica worked to break the habit of her helper and achiever patterns, and the more she calmed down her nervous system using meditation, the more she found her mood transforming. As she committed to cultivating a more sustainable and self-caring way of being, for the first time in many years she found herself feeling real happiness and joy once again.

And, as things really slowed down for Monica, she was also able to open to the deeper healing that really needed to happen in her heart. As we turn our attention toward this next step in your healing journey, we first need to put a spotlight on the ways you've learned to not feel your feelings.

CHAPTER 11

The Six Emotional Defenses

Lauren was in her late thirties and appeared to have an enviable life. Her home was a beautiful cottage in an idyllic village on the outskirts of London, and a Porsche, her pride and joy, sat in the driveway. She'd built a successful career which saw her travelling the world, and she was hoping to start a family with her boyfriend, adding to their already busy household of dogs and cats.

Only, things weren't quite as they seemed. Throughout her adult life, Lauren had struggled with depression, anxiety, and eating disorders. More recently, she'd also been experiencing crippling fatigue. The polished veneer she'd carefully constructed was starting to crack and, as is the case for most of us, the roots to it all lay in her childhood.

Lauren's mother had given birth to her in South Africa, but she'd quickly decided she couldn't cope, and put her up for adoption. At the last minute, Lauren's father decided he didn't want to lose his baby and brought her back to his home in England. For the first eight years of her life, Lauren was close to her father and stepmother, but then they had their own child together and suddenly, she was no longer made to feel welcome.

At the age of 10, Lauren was sent to live with her mother, who put constant pressure on her around how she looked, telling her to diet and lose weight.

Before long, Lauren was passed on again, this time sent to live with her aunt and uncle. This didn't last long, either, and in time Lauren's father and stepmother reluctantly took her back.

Lauren was constantly moving around; at one point she attended four schools in six months. Never staying in one location for more than a few years made it impossible to build sustainable friendships with other children. At the earliest opportunity, aged 16, Lauren left home, but her life didn't get any easier.

She self-funded her way through university, working three jobs while studying for her degree. Not surprisingly, she had a breakdown in her final year. As soon as she'd recovered some sense of normality, she threw herself headlong into her career. She believed that the more self-sufficient she was, the less dependent she'd be on others, and the safer she'd be in the world.

Emotional Self-harm

Lauren and I first started working together on my YouTube series *In Therapy with Alex Howard*, and I was struck immediately by the contrast between the self she showed to the world and how she felt on the inside. It reminded me that often, the more perfect our presented self-image, the greater the suffering and the more we're feeling the need to hide.

It was clear to me that for Lauren to heal the traumas of her past, she first had to be in contact with her emotional truth. The problem was that much of her adult life had been built around her strategies to not feel her emotions. Be it avoiding heartbreak at the end of a relationship by partying day and night or having breast implants and Botox injections to deal with her self-esteem issues, Lauren's solution to painful feelings was to do whatever she could to change them or avoid feeling them.

When the ultimate longing of our heart is for the love, safety, and boundaries we so desperately need, to spend our life constantly running from listening to these impulses is, in a sense, a form of self-harm. Although there are of course the obvious examples of self-harm, such as cutting and inflicting deliberate injury on the body, in my experience many of us unknowingly use much subtler forms. Anytime we reject the longing of our heart and ignore our core emotional needs, we're harming ourselves.

In many ways, Lauren's story is the story of all of us. As we've been exploring, when we don't digest and process our emotions, they don't just disappear. Indeed, the more intensely we suppress our emotions, the harder we must work to get away from them.

Ultimately, to heal our emotional trauma, we must be able to *feel* it. Put another way, you can't heal what you don't feel. By learning to turn toward and open to our emotions, we're taking an important step in not just healing the past but moving into a future free of our past sufferings.

Understanding the Six Emotional Defenses

Several years ago, as part of the Therapeutic Coaching® model, my colleague Anna Duschinsky and I mapped the different strategies we'd observed our patients (and ourselves!) using to avoid connecting with themselves emotionally. We call these 'the six emotional defenses,' as effectively they're six different ways we can defend against feeling our emotions. Put another way, they're six forms of self-harm, because they're ways of rejecting ourselves and our emotional experience.

By putting a spotlight on our emotional defenses and understanding them more deeply, we can begin to open up choices in our habits and behavior. Remember, if you can see it, you don't have to be it, and the more awareness we have, the more choices we give ourselves. It's worth noting that we can use one or all of the emotional defenses listed below at different points in our lives.

1. Avoidance and distraction – constantly staying busy and distracted from our emotions so we don't have time or space to feel them.

2. State changing – using external 'tools,' such as food, alcohol, drugs, and exercise to change how we feel.

3. Analysis – using our intellect and mind to 'think' about how we feel, instead of actually feeling.

4. Blaming others for our feelings – rather than feeling our feelings as our own, we blame others for our emotions and therefore don't fully experience them.

5. Empaths – feeling others' feelings as though they're our own emotions, which makes it hard to distinguish what we actually feel.

6. Somatizing – experiencing emotions as physical symptoms; for example, physical pain as a manifestation of unprocessed emotional pain.

Let's now look at these emotional defenses in some detail. As we do so, once again I'd like to encourage you to be gentle with yourself. This is delicate material and using it as ammunition to beat up on yourself isn't only unkind, it also adds more blocks to your healing.

1: Avoidance and Distraction

There are numerous different avoidance and distraction defenses we can use. From the subtle, such as always having the radio or TV on in the background, to the more blatant, such as working every minute of every day, so we don't have time to think, let alone feel. The core principle of this defense is that by filling our senses with noise in its many forms, we're able to keep our mind occupied and our attention away from our emotions.

The more intense the feelings we're trying to avoid and distract ourselves from, the more dramatic the strategies we might find ourselves using. For Lauren, the strategy was always being on the go, whether at work or play. In fact, she took pride in this, and her friends knew her for it. When she felt anxious, she'd busy herself more, and when her heart was telling her she needed time to feel, she'd push herself harder to get a promotion.

Do any of the following statements sound familiar to you?

- You're always busy and need to be on the go.

- You feel the need to always have some form of background noise, such as the TV or radio.

- You don't feel comfortable being quiet and alone with yourself – you always need some form of stimulation.

- You can't slow down and relax your body, or you only switch off when you're totally exhausted.

- You're constantly overcommitting to everyone in your life, except yourself.

2: State Changing

At its heart, state changing is using any kind of external 'tool' to change how we feel. Some of these tools may, on the surface, appear healthy and appropriate, while others might be much more harmful. The more obvious state-changing tools include sex, drugs, alcohol, and food. Some less obvious examples are exercise, seeking constant highs at work, and obsessive dating.

It's not that all these things are inherently wrong; the issue here is the way we obsessively use these tools to change how we feel. For example, going to the gym to blow off steam after a long day at work is entirely appropriate, and indeed it helps to shift our state in a positive way; however, being so obsessed with exercise that we use it to constantly get rid of our feelings is a form of self-rejection.

State changing is often used when someone has a lot of trauma or emotions that are simply too strong to avoid and distract from, and in a sense, it can be a form of self-medication. It can also play out in people who feel emotionally numb as a shutdown response to emotional, physical, or intellectual neglect, and want to just feel something.

Do any of the following statements sound familiar?

- You can only relax and unwind at the end of the day with several glasses of wine – physiologically needing a glass of wine to relax isn't the same as enjoying one from time to time.

- Whenever you feel emotional, you reach for food to change how you feel.

- You have a current issue with, or a history of, addiction to drugs, sex, alcohol, gambling, or something else that's potentially destructive.

- You're always chasing the next adventure and constantly looking to positive experiences in the future for something to make you feel better now.

3: Analysis

Overanalyzing and intellectualizing our feelings, rather than feeling them, is a way to believe that we're in touch with our emotions without actually being so. Often, there's a lot of mental activity, and when we're asked how we feel, we tend to instinctively reply with a response beginning, 'I think...'.

Analysis can be particularly tricky to spot, sometimes. On the surface, it can appear that we're in touch with our feelings because we may be able to describe them in surprisingly articulate ways. However, there's a big difference between being able to describe our feelings by thinking about them and actually feeling and surrendering to them.

Analysis is a common defense if we grew up in an environment that valued intellect over feelings. It's also often the result of there simply not being enough emotional safety to leave the apparent security of our mind in order to feel the movements of our heart.

As a result, we find ourselves constantly trying to *think* our way to a *feeling* of security. The belief is, *If I can just understand everything that's going on and have an answer to everything that might come up, I'll feel safe.* The problem is that the more we do this, the more we disconnect from our emotions. As I explained earlier, the sense of safety that we seek is a feeling not a thought, so no amount of thinking will ever get us there.

Part of the problem with analysis is that it drives a constant state of anxiety, and the more intense our emotions become, the faster our mind must go to escape them. It can also be a driver behind patterns such as obsessive-compulsive disorder (OCD), where we believe that our safety is the result of certain thoughts or actions.

Do any of the following statements sound familiar?

- You suffer from anxiety and an overactive mind.

- To feel safe, you need to assess situations in advance to understand what might happen.

- You find yourself describing how you feel in a cognitive way rather than feeling how you feel in your actual emotions.

- You believe that certain conditions need to be met for you to feel safe.

- You feel disconnected from the world emotionally and confused by other people's overemotional reactions.

4: Blaming Others for Our Feelings

This is where we're somewhat in touch with our feelings, but rather than actually feeling them, we instead get caught up in the story of why they're other people's fault and place the blame on them. We can end up feeling a lot without ever fully being in touch with it or processing our emotions.

Perhaps you're constantly angry at your parents, who you feel failed you as a child; or maybe you're easily triggered by others' behavior and are quick to blame them for how you feel. Or maybe you feel a constant sense of righteousness about world events and those greedy and dishonest people you believe are the cause of everyone else's misery.

Of course, what's rather interesting is that those same instincts of greed and dishonesty exist in us all. And, although I'm not here to defend the actions of many of those in power, and it's certainly true that privilege exists and the world isn't an even playing field, if a primary force in our psyche is a constant blaming of others, the danger is that we become trapped in a cycle of reactivity, which robs us of the opportunity to go deeper into our own heart.

Do any of the following statements sound familiar?

- You react abruptly and harshly to other people's actions.

- You're quick to criticize and blame others for making you feel something.

- You find yourself regularly ranting in your mind about how others have behaved.

5: Empaths

Empaths, sometimes known as 'highly sensitive people,' take on the feelings of others and experience them as their own. They can be highly sensitive to the environment they're in and the people they're around. Being an empath can be exhausting and further add to our seemingly never-ending emotional load.

With the other emotional defenses, the issue can be that we're not feeling much at all, but empaths have the opposite problem – they're feeling so much that they're overwhelmed. And because much of what they're feeling isn't even their 'stuff,' it's hard for them to separate their emotions from those of others, or to even get through others' 'stuff' in order to process their own.

Indeed, part of the challenge for empaths is that although they feel as if they're in touch with their emotions because of all that they're feeling, often what they're doing is carrying others' emotions for them, creating even more distance from their own. And, although in that moment it can seem that they're gifting someone a huge emotional service by holding their emotions for them, in truth no one can metabolize another person's emotions. So, it's a fruitless pursuit, even if the empath's intentions are good.

To be clear, I'm not saying we shouldn't hold space for other people or open our heart to their pain and suffering. My point is that by actually feeling and taking on others' emotions, we don't serve them, and ultimately, we may be falling under the spell of a familiar pattern for ourselves.

Being an empath can be a product of growing up in an environment that felt unsafe, and in which we learned to navigate by merging with and feeling other people's emotions in a bid to predict or control their behavior to keep them safe. It can also be the result of growing up in an environment where there wasn't a lot of space for your feelings, such as being a second or third child with emotionally dominating siblings.

Do any of the following statements sound familiar?

- You find being around other people exhausting.

- You're more in touch with other people's feelings than they are.

- Other people find you a soothing and supporting presence to be around and often report feeling 'lighter' after being with you.

- The world can feel like an overwhelming and emotionally intense place to be.

- You notice that you attract people into your life who are emotionally needy and not good at expressing their own emotions in a healthy way.

6: Somatizing

Somatizing is where we experience our emotions as physical symptoms. Put simply, our unprocessed emotional pain becomes physical pain. The energy of our emotions must go somewhere in our body, and physical symptoms are a way of expressing it. The problem is, this doesn't help us to process the emotional pain, and it causes more suffering along the way.

Physical symptoms can be almost anything, but particularly common are digestive issues, back pain, and headaches. Over the years, there have been various models that track emotional issues to physical symptoms, and although I think these can sometimes be a useful source of reflection, I've never found them particularly accurate, as in my experience everyone's unique in the way they store and hold their emotions.

It's also important to note that somatizing alone may not be the only cause of a symptom. For example, there may also be a physical issue; however, somatizing emotions either adds to this load or inhibits the body's natural healing capacity.

Do any of the following statements sound familiar?

- You experience digestive problems.

- You suffer from chronic pain without a known physical origin.

- You have migraines.

- You have unexplained physical symptoms.

- Your physical symptoms worsen when you feel overwhelmed.

- When you're more relaxed, you sometimes notice an improvement in your physical symptoms.

As you reflect on these six emotional defenses, which of them feel the most familiar to you? As I said earlier, you may well experience several or indeed all of them. And remember, it isn't that they're all necessarily wrong. The problems come when we use them as ongoing ways of disconnecting from, defending against, and ultimately not feeling and healing our emotions.

Uncover Your Emotional Defenses

The more awareness we have of these emotional defenses, the more we're able to make different and healthier choices. Often, awareness of them alone will be a helpful step toward changing them. It's worth noting that awareness of our defenses tends to evolve in three stages:

- We recognize that this is a defense we have, but without specific examples.

- We can come up with specific examples of the defense and see how it plays out.

- We can see the defense in real time, as it happens.

As we move to seeing these emotional defenses in real time, we're empowered to change them. So, the purpose of these three stages is to become better at recognizing the defenses, with specific examples of them in hindsight, and then ultimately to see them as they happen.

Situation | Feeling | Response

This exercise is designed to help you uncover the emotional defenses you use in your life. I encourage you to do it daily for a week or two, ideally at the end of the day, to enable you to identify examples. The steps are very simple, but also very powerful. You can download a worksheet to help you complete the exercise at www.alexhoward.com/trauma.

1. The first thing you're looking for is a **situation** where something happened that triggered (or could have triggered) an emotional response. This could have been an altercation with your boss, dropping your breakfast on the floor, being late to meet a friend, or pretty much anything else.

2. Next, you're looking for what you were **feeling**. Now, in reality, your emotional defense might have kicked in so quickly that you didn't get a chance to feel it. Indeed, the reason why you're doing this exercise is to understand how you distract yourself from the way you feel. So, if you don't know what you felt in the situation, you can have a guess at what it might have been.

3. Finally, we're looking for your **response** to your feeling. What did you do with how you felt? Did you avoid it? Did you look for a way to change your feeling? Did you rationalize your feeling away? Did you blame someone else for your feeling? Did you become consumed by how someone else was feeling? Did you develop a physical symptom, such as a headache? In other words, what **emotional defense** did you use?

Here's an example:

- **Situation**: While you were having dinner with a family member, they criticized you for something you'd said in all innocence.

- **Feeling**: You felt hurt, judged, and emotionally manipulated.

- **Response**: You started speaking more quickly to try and distract yourself. You also ate more food than you wanted to as a way of trying to change the way you felt. And as you were driving home, you noticed you had a headache.

- **Emotional defenses**: Avoidance and distraction (speaking more quickly); state changing (overeating); somatizing (headache).

By doing this exercise regularly, you'll likely notice which emotional defenses you consistently use. Remember, this knowledge is power. And once we've looked at how you can actually *feel* your feelings in the next few chapters, you'll have a whole set of powerful new choices.

Healing Is Possible

Returning to Lauren once last time, as she and I worked through her emotional defenses, she had several significant insights, and she also found the process liberating. Although it was hard to acknowledge to herself just how much she'd been escaping her feelings over the years, it was a huge relief to realize that there was another way to behave.

Over several months, she made much more space in her life for herself, which included ending her toxic relationship, temporarily reducing her hours at work, and committing to her own healing. In time, she fundamentally changed her way of relating to herself and others and her health issues also started to transform.

Lauren also discovered that ultimately, feeling our emotions hurts so much less than rejecting them and constantly running away from them. Indeed, this is our next point of reflection together.

CHAPTER 12

Inquire Into Your Emotions

A s I settled into my comfortable chair at the Everyman Cinema in North London, I thought I was on a regular evening out with Tania (who at the time, was my relatively newfound love). I hadn't paid much attention to the movie we'd chosen; I was just happy to be out of the office early and relaxing.

We found ourselves watching Danny Boyle's film *127 Hours*, which is based on the true story of Aron Ralston, an experienced mountain climber who on a hiking trip in the USA, became trapped alone in a canyon with his lower right arm and hand crushed beneath a boulder. As the film unfolded, we witnessed his emotionally intense and deeply challenging attempts to escape over five excruciating days.

First, Aron attempted to free his arm using brute force, and when that failed, he tried screaming for help. As the hours passed, he went through every emotion possible, oscillating between hope, despair, and terror. Then, after several days without success, he gave up and resigned himself to certain death. In accepting the painful inevitability of his premature demise, he could at least finally surrender. He recorded goodbye messages to his loved ones on his video camera, carved RIP into the boulder, and succumbed to sleep.

When he woke up the following morning it slowly dawned on him that even praying for death was fruitless, because there he was, still trapped, in pain, and facing a very slow and painful dying process.

Eventually, he realized there was only one choice remaining. To free himself, he'd have to cut off his own arm. First, he had to snap his bones, and then, using the only tool he had, which was a blunt multi-purpose penknife, he cut through his skin before using the pliers on the penknife to cut through his tendons.

Following the Thread

Throughout the film, I was captivated by what I was seeing, and unaware that anything untoward was happening to me. That was, until the film ended, and I started crying. At this point in my life, I was relatively comfortable with my emotions, and I knew there was nothing to do but let the tears come.

As the credits rolled, however, my tears didn't quieten and pass as I'd expected. In fact, they started to intensify. Unfortunately, I'm not an elegant crier, but more of a snotty and spluttery one, so I'm sure those around me must have wondered what the hell was going on. Tania sweetly held my arm, and asked if I was OK, but I couldn't speak. I just nodded as the tears continued to engulf me. I couldn't move, but I also couldn't stop crying.

Thankfully, we'd parked around the corner from the cinema, and Tania held my hand as we walked quickly to the car, which to me suddenly seemed like a sanctuary of safety. There, I handed Tania the keys, nodding that she should drive, and once I'd slipped into the passenger seat, the tidal wave of emotion crashed through me again and the tears started flooding uncontrollably. Thankfully, Tania's training as a psychotherapist meant she knew she had to just sit with me and patiently hold the space while the emotion continued to release.

After at least another 10 minutes, I finally managed to get my breath a little. We'd planned to have dinner at one of our favorite restaurants, but Tania gently looked at me and said, 'Would you like to eat at home?' I simply nodded. As Tania drove, I gradually managed to find some space underneath the tears. As I'd learned to do over the years, I worked to tune in to what I was really feeling and to follow the thread in my own life to what had been triggered. It didn't take long for the answer to come.

Although the external events were very different, the inner journey that Aron had been on almost perfectly paralleled my emotional experience of being chronically ill with ME/CFS – the desperation and false hope; the rage and frustration; the grief and hopelessness. But what had really hit me was the terrible truth that even giving up didn't work because, just like Aron, I'd given up so many times, and yet the next morning I'd wake up and have to survive another day of my personal living hell. It also deeply moved me to see Aron finally find help and realize that he'd survived and was no longer alone.

For me, the experience of being trapped in a broken body that wouldn't heal, feeling utterly hopeless and alone, and the belief that I'd never get out was clearly a deep injury in my emotional body that hadn't yet fully healed. Witnessing Aron's journey had activated the unhealed memory of those same emotions inside my own heart and body. My big black sack of unprocessed emotions had opened and revealed a trauma that was ready to heal.

Later, as we sat in our kitchen, I shared what was coming up, and felt Tania's sweet and beautiful support and holding as she witnessed the spontaneous healing that had been triggered inside me. She knew there was nothing to be done but feel and welcome the feelings as they metabolized and processed.

The Tool of Inquiry

As we discussed earlier, mainstream psychology has been rather quick to dismiss our emotions as something to be fixed, ideally, or at least managed. However, the reality is that our emotional body, the home of our emotional life, needs nurturing and caring for just as much as our physical body does.

Our emotional body is often seen as a problematic or dysfunctional part of us that we should do our best to keep in check. And yet, in truth there's an incredible wisdom in the way we learn to suppress and lock away what's too difficult to feel at the time, and equally to be able to heal it at any point in the future when the conditions are right.

However, although our emotional body protects us at the time, unless we commit to making the space to ultimately feel the emotions it's locked way, we pay the price of being imprisoned by it for life.

We all have a dynamic universe of emotional experience living inside us, and for our trauma healing to happen we must learn to open to it. The question isn't whether we have emotions, it's how closely we're in touch with them. As we explored in the last chapter, we can have all kinds of defenses against feeling our emotions, but this doesn't mean they go away – instead, we have to run away from ourselves.

As we explored in Chapter 6, we develop a variety of beliefs and meanings about our emotions, which is how we manage to keep ourselves disconnected from feeling them. It's now time to begin to feel into what happens if we go beyond these beliefs. To do this, we're going to use a tool called Therapeutic Inquiry.

Going Beneath the Surface

The practice of Therapeutic Inquiry involves opening to and exploring our inner world and what's happening within it. With patience and skill, we learn to navigate and make sense of our inner universe, and in the process, we lay the foundation for our healing to happen. A metaphor I find helpful is that Therapeutic Inquiry is like finding our way through a pitch-black building guided only by a piece of thread. By staying quiet and connected to our experience, we can gently feel the next step, trusting that following the thread will take us where we need to go.

A simple example of Therapeutic Inquiry in action is my experience of watching the film *127 Hours*. By tuning in to how I was feeling, I was able to follow the thread to understand the origins and history beneath the emotions. What might appear to have been an extreme reaction to a well-made film, was in fact the gateway to accessing a deep potential for healing inside of me.

Inquiry can be used in this way retrospectively to make sense of something we're already feeling, but it can also be a powerful way of opening up and starting to feel emotions that are currently outside our conscious awareness.

Let's say you arrive home from work and are feeling on edge and slightly irritable. You take a bath, and as you are finally able to relax, you decide to inquire into what's going on. As you take some deep breaths into your feeling of irritability, beneath it you find a quite intense anxiety in your chest. As you give some space to the anxiety, in your mind you're curious as to what's *really* going on. By inviting the feeling and being steadfast in your attention toward it and encouraging a sense of safety while meeting the feeling from a loving place, you notice that the anxiety relaxes and reveals a feeling of sadness.

Deepening your connection with the feeling of sadness, you let the tears come and feel a sense of relief in your body for doing so. As you stay curious and open to your experience, memories appear in your mind of a close friend who passed away a few months ago. As you reflect on those memories, your heart feels soft and tender, and you realize how much you miss your friend.

Discover What's Really Going On

Here, your surface-level feeling of irritability was in fact a sign that you were out of touch with some important emotions that needed to be given space and loving attention. The feelings of sadness and loss don't need you to *do* anything; instead, they need you to *be* with them and give them some space. As you allow yourself to do so, you feel a warmth and love in your heart for your friend, and although you feel the loss, you also feel the love.

On reflection, you realize that your irritability was quite the opposite of something to be avoided or distracted from – it was a sign that you need to connect and be closer to yourself. In doing so, you're giving yourself the love and holding that you need and deserve. In a sense you're becoming the patient and attentive parent you perhaps always longed for.

If you reflect on the above example, you'll see that what you thought was going on at the surface level of your experience wasn't what was *really* going on. In fact, it was just a reaction to it and a way of avoiding it. This is so often the case in life. There's the surface level and then there's the deep level of what's really going on. The practice of Therapeutic Inquiry supports us in going beneath the surface level and following the thread to our deeper emotional experience, which is where our healing can really happen.

The surface level of our experience is so often what causes the suffering in our lives. Not only do we have to live with difficult emotions like anxiety, irritability, and frustration, but those around us must also live with us reacting from the place of these emotions. Furthermore, the life choices we tend to make from this place tend to be poor and perpetuate our own suffering.

Disconnection Feeds Disconnection

In my own life, one helpful realization I had is that when I'm disconnected from myself (i.e., living on the surface level of my emotions), I tend to make choices that support further disconnection. Put another way, disconnection feeds disconnection.

Let's take our example above, but have it play out another way. You get home from work and you're feeling the same irritability. Instead of choosing to take a bath, relax, and feel into your feelings, you head straight for the sofa and switch on the TV. While watching a show, you're also scrolling through social media on your phone.

As you spend the evening in a state of emotional disconnect, you find yourself making poor nutritional choices for dinner, and consume this food without enough time to chew it and give your digestive system a chance to properly metabolize it.

Fueled by the stimulation of social media, the fast-paced TV series you're bingeing, and the pumping cortisol you've just triggered by the meal of negative nutrition (food that takes more energy to digest than it gives you), you're nicely protected from feeling any of your emotions. Ultimately, your disconnection just fed more disconnection.

However, just as disconnection feeds disconnection, connection also feeds connection. Taking the original example, having got closer to how you really feel, the chances are you'll make some different choices that evening. Perhaps you'll reach out to other friends and share your feelings, or perhaps you'll just go gently to stay closer to yourself.

The Three Centers of Therapeutic Inquiry

Therapeutic Inquiry can happen from three different centers inside you, and each has something to bring to the practice. You can inquire from your mind, your heart, and your body. Let's explore each of these now.

1: Mind

The gift our mind offers to the practice of inquiry is our ability to observe what's happening, make connections between different elements, and in time penetrate the details with our awareness. However, if our inquiry becomes a cognitive exercise on its own, it will go nowhere, as ultimately, we're seeking to move beyond our mind. Also, we must be careful not to get caught in analysis paralysis, which is where we do a lot of analyzing and thinking about our emotions instead of actually feeling them.

2: Heart

Ultimately, inquiry is a practice of the heart. We're tuning in to and listening to our emotions and feelings about what's happening. By meeting our inquiry from our heart, we're also bringing a quality of love and softness that helps build the inner trust and openness that's so important. However, if we're only using our heart, we can find ourselves lost in a sea of emotion without the ability to reflect and understand what's happening, which is why our mind is also important.

3: Body

Inquiry is a practice that happens in our body. As you did with the meditation practice in Chapter 9, you're learning to soften your mental attention, relax, and come home to the experience of your body. It's easy to think of the body as a lump of meat and bones that has no inherent intelligence, but the reality is quite the opposite.

So much of the wisdom we're trying to contact and unlock lives in our body, and a key part of our inquiry practice is to open to and welcome this wisdom. While our heart is the home of our emotions, our body is the realm of sensations and feelings. By learning to tune in to these, we can use them as a guide along our journey of inquiry.

We all come to the practice of inquiry with our own areas of comfort, and the places we need to grow and develop. Perhaps you have a sharp and inquisitive mind but approach your body with a closed heart. Or perhaps you're good at feeling your emotions but you get lost in them and need to become more skilled at grounding yourself in the immediate experience of your bodily sensations. The key is to develop the areas we're less experienced in while being guided by the gifts we already have at our disposal.

Who's Driving Your Inquiry?

The essence of inquiry is that we're moving beyond our known experience and allowing our truth in that moment to reveal itself. Inquiry isn't about attempting to confirm what we already know to be true – it's about discovering what's beneath our surface-level understanding and what's happening in our deeper experience.

To do this, of course, we need to have the ability to self-regulate our nervous system and build an inner sense of safety, and to encourage our experience to continue to reveal itself from a place of love and gentleness. If we're attempting to control our experience and rejecting or controlling what's happening, our nervous system will shut down instead of opening up.

Your Therapeutic Inquiry Practice

Now that we've looked at the key places from which you're meeting your inner experience of inquiry, it's time to explore the steps of Therapeutic Inquiry.

1. Find a quiet place where you won't be disturbed.

2. Relax into your inner experience – starting with a period of meditation is often helpful.

3. Explore. What are you feeling right now? What do you feel in your body? Which emotions are there? What's going through your mind?

4. Allow yourself to open up to how you feel and see what happens when you relax more deeply into it.

5. When you feel deeper into your experience, what opens up next? Where does the thread of inquiry take you? See if you can follow the thread rather than trying to direct it.

6. If you get lost at any point, just bring your attention to your breath and sensing your body and explore what's there now.

There are no right and wrong ways to inquire. What's important is giving space to the truth of how you feel. The gift of inquiry is that you learn to have a new relationship with both your emotions as they are now and your emotional history. So much of what we experience in our lives isn't about what's happening today but about our emotional history, which we still need to process. The more we do so, the more we're able to respond freely and proportionately to our day-to-day life experiences.

My hope for you is that Therapeutic Inquiry will become a daily practice that will not only help you to heal your past but also enable you to make sense of your present and avoid it storing up more unprocessed traumas. As you integrate inquiry into your daily life, I think you'll notice a lot more emotional space opening up. However, what can often also happen is that we hit inner resistance, and this is what we're going to tackle in the next chapter.

CHAPTER 13

Moving Beyond Inner Resistance

Coming to therapy wasn't Daryl's own idea. In fact, a polite way of putting it is that he'd been strongly encouraged to do so by his girlfriend, but I believe there was an implicit ultimatum – he had to find a way to moderate his drinking, or their relationship would be over.

Daryl was in his late twenties and worked as a tradesman, but he aspired to become a property developer. He told me that he'd enjoyed a drink since first tasting alcohol as a teenager, but the problem was that drinking had become more than just a way to wind down at the end of a hard day's work.

Daryl drank every day. On weekends, he'd start at lunchtime, with barely a pause before he virtually collapsed in the early hours. Like many people who've become dependent on alcohol, Daryl was convinced he wasn't an alcoholic. Only, now that he wanted to control his drinking, he found he couldn't, and it was starting to frighten him. Time and again he'd had the best of intentions to stop, and he considered himself a determined person in other areas of his life, but it wasn't working. It pained him to admit it, but he needed help.

As we explored some of Daryl's emotional history, I saw that he was using alcohol as a way of self-medicating his emotions. As I asked him about his childhood and what was happening around the time he'd started drinking, he somewhat reluctantly told me about the tragic loss of his mother.

When Daryl was 16, his mother was diagnosed with bowel cancer, which then quickly spread. Despite her determined efforts to fight it, she'd died just nine months later. Daryl told me that he'd been in shock initially, but then he'd just 'dealt with it' and got on with his life. His father had been in and out of prison over the years, and even when he was around, he'd been an unhelpful influence, to say the least. After Daryl lost his mum, his father told him that he was a man now and he therefore didn't need a mother.

A Layer of Defense

When I suggested to Daryl that his drinking might be related to the loss of his mother, he looked at me with a confused expression. 'Shit happens, and you deal with it,' he said. To which I replied, 'Yes, Daryl, shit does happen, but I don't think you *have* dealt with it.' Thankfully, I'd built a good connection with him by this point and so he pondered my words for long enough to recognize there might be some truth in them.

In essence, Daryl had learned to lock away his emotions and disconnect from his emotional body. Drinking alcohol helped him to continue to numb himself to his feelings, and his unconscious fear was that if he went too long without his drug of choice, he'd start to feel again.

Over the next few sessions, I worked with Daryl to build some awareness of his other emotional defenses, which included analyzing rather than feeling and blaming others for the way he was feeling. We then started to work experientially to inquire into what he was feeling in the moment. But as we did so, he'd consistently come up with responses along the lines of,

'I don't feel anything.' Ultimately, the same inner resistance that had been there when his mother died when he was 16, was still protecting him from feeling his emotions.

For Daryl, this inner resistance showed up as an emptiness when he tried to feel his emotions. For others it might be a feeling of anger or wanting to push away, or an over-intellectualizing in their mind. Whichever way it shows up, though, it's a layer of defense against feeling our emotions.

Inner resistance is our emotional body's intelligent way of protecting us from feelings that we didn't have the resources to feel at the time. It was likely not just the only response available to us but also genuinely the best option we had. And it worked because here we are to tell the story (and to create a new one going forward).

In a sense, the breakthrough at one stage becomes the limitation at the next. The same strategy that was crucial to our survival is now the very thing in the way of our moving forward. The walls that once kept us safe are now keeping us trapped. And as much as they might now frustrate us, we must treat those walls carefully and with great respect.

When our emotional defenses work to protect us, it's rarely effective to try and smash them down. Indeed, the harder we push against them, the stronger they become in pushing back because that's what they've learned to do. What we resist will persist.

Learning to Meet Your Emotional Needs

To loosen the grip that our inner resistance has on our emotional life, we can't meet it from a place of harshness and pushing. In fact, what we need is the opposite. The antidote to our inner shutdown is to give ourselves the qualities whose absence caused us to shut down in the first place.

Ultimately, we must learn to meet our three core emotional needs of boundaries, safety, and love, as doing so will provide the key to unlock our walls of defense. So, take some time now to learn how you can more effectively meet your core emotional needs.

Creating Inner Boundaries

Developing inner boundaries is ultimately about learning to be steady and steadfast with our experience. It's being strong enough to keep our attention and presence with our difficult emotions. Just as a skillful therapist stays attentive and present to a client's difficult emotions, we need to learn to do the same for ourselves.

Think about a small child who's upset about something; the message they need from their caregiver is that they're OK, and what they're feeling is OK. The way the child receives this message is driven by how their caregiver responds to their emotions. Do they try and shut them down, or do they pull away when the child expresses them? Or do they encourage the child and lean in with the wish to hear more when they open up?

To create a safe space for your emotions to move and flow, you need to meet them from an encouraging place that says they're welcome and OK. Put another way, your inner boundary that meets your emotions invites them in and makes space for them. The way to do this is to notice your direct response to your feelings when they arise.

I often ask my clients, 'How do you feel about how you feel?' When I was working with Daryl, what he felt was emptiness, and how he felt about this was irritated and annoyed. Ultimately, he thought he should be feeling something, and so the place where he met the emptiness was one of rejection. Meeting his absence of emotion from this place of rejection just deepened the inner shutdown and protection. As we worked to soften his inner emotional boundary and bring in some more gentleness and curiosity, things started to open a little.

Creating Inner Safety

Another key reason why we defend against and shut down our emotions is because we've learned it isn't safe to feel them. If you think back to my story of witnessing my sister's destructive use of her own emotions, you'll recall that I learned that feeling emotions was a dangerous thing. As we discussed earlier, as children we're dependent on our primary caregivers to co-regulate their nervous system with our own, teaching our system that we're safe and that it's OK to feel. As adults, we need to learn to self-regulate our nervous system to build our own sense of inner safety.

This is where meditation practice (see Chapter 9) is particularly important. By learning to regulate our nervous system and stay present to our experience, even if it feels difficult, we're sending the message that we're safe. This creates enough relaxation for our feelings to start to open.

Creating Inner Love

While our inner boundaries and safety create the environment for our inner defenses to soften and our emotions to open, it's the quality of love that draws them out. It's the curiosity and warmth of our love that allows emotions to express themselves and the process of healing to begin. It's the quality of love that says we're perfect just as we are, that our emotions are valid and deserve to be felt. Like a loving and attentive mother adoring a child, we're meeting our emotions from a true place of acceptance.

The kind of love we express to our emotions and their defenses is also important. It isn't a conditional love where some emotions are welcome, and others are not. The key is that whatever we're experiencing isn't only welcome, we're truly interested in it.

Open Your Emotions

The purpose of this exercise is to practice softening your emotional defenses and inviting your emotions to open. This can take some time because you're breaking an existing habit and working to create a new inner landscape of openness.

1. Find a quiet place where you won't be disturbed and start with a few minutes of meditation.

2. Notice how you feel. Do you feel a particular emotion, or do you feel nothing?

3. Explore how you're feeling toward your feelings (or lack of). Do you feel open toward your feelings, or is there a sense of rejection or pulling away?

4. Practice softening your inner boundary with your feelings and tell them, inside your mind, that they're welcome.

5. Use the quiet attention that meditation brings to self-regulate your nervous system and build a sense of inner safety that your feelings are safe.

6. See what happens when you bring a quality of love toward your emotions, expressing sincere interest and curiosity in them.

7. If your emotions start to open and flow, give them space, welcome them, and relax into the experience. If they don't, be gentle with that as well.

This is an exercise you can do reactively if you feel emotionally triggered by something, and proactively on its own each day. It'll work particularly well when done immediately after your meditation practice.

Let Go, Let the Emotions Flow

With the previous exercise and what we've been building up to in the last few chapters, we're ultimately creating an inner state of emotional movement. We need to let go and let the emotions flow. By understanding the strategies that we use to emotionally disconnect, by inquiring into our immediate experience, and by relaxing our inner defenses, we can allow our emotions to have the space they need to process.

Remember, we're wired to heal, and our emotional body can heal itself, given the right environment, just as our physical body does. What you're learning to do here is create the inner environment that allows the healing to happen. And when it does, your whole world can start to change.

You may recall the story of my own emotional opening, at the beginning of the book; I wrestled with it, my inner resistance and defenses holding on. But once I took the leap, everything became easier. We might start feeling a lot more, but it hurts us a lot less.

What this will probably look like is our emotions starting to open up. We might feel any number of emotions – including anger and intense sadness – or we might just have the sensation of energy moving inside us. The key here is that we're learning to allow the emotions to flow and move; in a sense, we're emptying that black sack of old, unprocessed emotions we carry around with us.

To be clear, though, we're not talking about throwing these emotions at other people, as this will likely cause more suffering and pain for everyone, including ourselves. We want to let the energy flow out of us, but not all over others.

You may find that the instructions I've given in this chapter are enough for you to do this work by yourself, but some people will need holding and support from others, such as a qualified therapist. This is especially true when the events of our trauma were particularly overwhelming. In such instances, additional processing tools, such as Eye Movement Desensitization and Reprocessing (EMDR) and Emotional Freedom Technique (EFT/Tapping) can be immensely helpful.

The Layers of Our Emotions

As your emotions start to open, you may find they're like the layers of an onion. Under each layer, there's another one waiting to reveal itself. Indeed, there's often a wisdom to the way our emotions protect and reveal each other as we open to them. We're all different in our emotional experience, but there's a particular sequence I commonly see:

1. Anxiety/fear

2. Anger/hatred

3. Sadness/longing

4. Deep connection

If we look at why this might be the case, it makes sense that the surface-level emotions are anxiety and fear – this may be our maladaptive stress response and our nervous system running quickly to draw us into our head and away from the feeling. As we move beyond this, we reveal feelings such as anger and hatred, which allow us to feel ready for action and to protect against the more vulnerable feelings underneath.

As we process the anger and hatred, we can then more fully surrender to the feeling of collapse that may exist underneath it. This is the realm of our sadness and longing. But ultimately, our emotions are never a bottomless pit, and when we have the courage to allow them to open and free themselves, the reward is a deep sense of relief and connection to ourselves. The more we liberate our emotions, the more we liberate our true self.

And although superficially it can sound like semantics, it's often helpful to get as specific as we can in naming the emotions we're feeling. For example, there's a significant difference in the felt sense between anger and hatred. Anger feels fiery and as if we want to have a fight whereas hatred is cold, calculating, and much more precise in its actions.

I notice that often when someone can find the right name for the emotion they're experiencing, it allows them to feel into it and welcome it more fully. And when we've been out of touch with our emotions for a long time, finding the correct words can be tricky. Just as we do when learning a new language, we need to become familiar with the vocabulary.

What Does Emotional Healing Look Like?

At this point, you might be wondering whether I advocate a world in which we're all feeling *everything*, fully, all the time, in all situations. Let me be super clear: *I do not.* Our emotional defenses didn't happen by accident; they have their place, and what's appropriate in one situation may well not be in another.

Furthermore, to reiterate something I said earlier, I'm not suggesting we should just throw whatever we're feeling at whoever's closest to us. This is not only childish, but it also often causes even more suffering for everyone. What we're talking about is a healthy and mature relationship with our feelings, one in which we're taking the time to process and heal our past by working through the excess baggage in our metaphorical black sack. At the same time, we're also learning to live more fully in the present moment and to unlock a future that isn't limited by the negative impacts of our past.

But what does healthy emotional healing look like? To those who don't know us particularly well, it may seem that nothing's really changing in the short term – we're just a little more sensitive and reflective, perhaps. But those closer to us may notice that we're feeling a lot more. And at times, in the quiet of our own mind, we may find ourselves wondering what the hell we've got ourselves into while we're playing emotional catch-up!

If we're spending a lot of time around the people who played a significant role in setting up our trauma ECHOs, we may also find that we need a little more space from them in the short term. We'll talk more about how to manage these relationships in Part III.

Another dynamic that can be particularly tricky to manage while we're working to open ourselves more emotionally is that we become more critical of ourselves. In a sense, the inner voice that's worked hard to keep everything in check can get rather vocal when we shake things up in our inner world. We'll get to this in the next chapter.

Breaking the Pattern

Returning to Daryl's story, as we worked together to change his relationship with his emotions, gradually cultivating an inner space of boundaries, safety, and love, initially he reported feeling a little more sensitive and reactive but not much else; however, he stayed with it.

One day he had a conversation with his girlfriend in which she asked him about his mother. As he responded, seemingly (to him) out of nowhere, he began to cry. Reflecting on this experience in our next session, Daryl said that his instinct had been to shut down, but the work we'd been doing allowed him to open up instead, and before he knew it, the floodgates had opened, and he cried for almost an hour straight.

From this point on, Daryl found it so much easier to engage in his therapy. He worked through his sadness at the loss of his mother and through the intense rage and hatred he felt for his father, which in time, opened to a place of longing for his love and care. Over the months that we worked together, Daryl gradually noticed that he was drinking less, and we added in some additional pattern-breaking techniques (including those in Chapter 10). In one of our final sessions, Daryl walked in and told me that he'd gone an entire weekend without a drink, including attending a friend's wedding where he'd been the only guest not drinking. I can remember the look of pride on his face like it was yesterday.

A year or so after I finished working with Daryl, I received a moving email in which he told me that his girlfriend was pregnant, and they were engaged. Recalling something I'd said in one of our sessions, the final line of the message was, 'It's time to break the cycle of emotional neglect from fathers in my family.'

CHAPTER 14
Transform Your Inner Critic

Beverley appeared to have had a happy and loving upbringing. A single child, she'd spent a great deal of time with her mother and was always immaculately turned out. However, as is often the case in families, things were not as they seemed.

Beverley's mother had suffered from severe anxiety, and she saw her daughter as her comfort and an extension of her own needs. What Beverley needed or wanted was of no importance; indeed, the parent–child relationship was effectively reversed, and Beverley was there to take care of and meet the needs of her mother.

As we unpacked her childhood together while filming my *In Therapy with Alex Howard* series, Beverley shared one particularly striking event that occurred when she was around 11 years old. Her mother had asked her what she'd like to eat for her evening meal, adding that she could have whatever she wanted. This never happened: Beverley's mother liked sweet food, and so that was what she fed her daughter, whether she liked it or not.

Now, most children given this choice would likely opt for ice cream or chocolate, and if they had to have something savory it would involve fries and plenty of tomato ketchup (or perhaps that's just my kids!). Not

Beverley: She was desperate for a proper meal and so she asked for meat and vegetables.

Beverley's mother responded to this request with irritation, annoyed that she'd have to go find the ingredients and spend time cooking. She'd assumed that Beverley would choose a dish that she would want – the idea that her daughter might have different preferences wasn't even in her world of possibility.

A few months after this incident, Beverley had a nervous breakdown and became entirely unable to function. Although as a teenager she'd worked hard to get things back on track, and when she was in her twenties, and at other times later, she'd put herself through therapy, for much of her life she'd struggled with intimate relationships and had suicidal thoughts.

The Inner Critic in Action

At the time I met her, Beverley had recently retired after a 40-year career as a dentist and was feeling somewhat lost; she was unsure of her purpose in life and wanted to heal and make sense of her past. As we uncovered more of the pieces of her trauma jigsaw, the events of her life increasingly made sense. Indeed, the intense love deficit she'd grown up with had spilled into everything, from her relationships and friendships to her health.

At the heart of many of Beverley's struggles was the way she spoke to herself. This inner voice, or inner critic (more on this coming up), is shaped by the way our primary caregivers spoke to us and treated us, and with her mother having been so harsh with her, Beverley developed a particularly vicious and cruel inner critic.

To her inner critic, whatever Beverley did was wrong, and it would also regularly imagine the cruel and unkind things it was convinced others were thinking and saying about her. This constant internal abuse made it particularly difficult for Beverley to make big life decisions, and to reach out and build the friendships and connections that she needed and deserved.

How Do You Speak to Yourself?

Sigmund Freud (whose work we touched on in Chapter 6) was a fascinating character who was mapping human psychology in the late 19th century, an era of significant sexual repression, and as a result, one must hold some of his theories in this context to understand why be believed that repressed sexual desires and impulses are behind most human behavior.

However, one of Freud's immensely valuable contributions to psychology was his concepts of the id, the ego, and the superego of the human personality. The superego is the part of the mind whose job it is to keep the more unruly areas of our psyche in check. In Freud's native tongue, German, the superego is the 'über ich,' meaning 'over I.' Effectively, it's our internal voice of judgement, which sits above us and judges, criticizes, and directs our inner world, our choices, and our behaviors. It's this voice that constantly tells us that we are broken and that our suffering is our own fault.

In popular psychology, we refer to this personality structure as our inner critic, as effectively it's that voice inside us all that's endlessly criticizing and judging us. For some, this voice is subtle and quiet, while for others it's raging and unavoidable.

One of the significant impacts of our trauma is that we become normalized to talking to ourselves in abusive, harsh, and ultimately unhelpful ways. As we work to reset our nervous system and heal our trauma, we must ensure that this ultimately translates to a new way of relating to ourselves. To do this, we need to work on transforming our inner critic; if we don't, we'll continue the cycle of trauma in the way we treat ourselves.

I think that the damaging impact the inner critic has on our life cannot be overstated. From influencing our basic mood from day to day, to limiting our capacity to pursue the things we're passionate about, to being part of the makeup of our inner resistance to feeling our emotions, when our inner critic is at work, it affects how we feel. The inner critic constantly drains our energy, which means we end up fulfilling significantly less of our true potential in the world.

Don't We Need Our Inner Critic?

At this point you might be thinking, *OK, I recognize that I have this voice, but surely, I need it to function in the world. Without it I'd have no sense of morals or right and wrong.* To which I'd respond: It's true that as children we do need this inner voice because it helps keep a version of our parents present when we're alone, and it helps us learn how to navigate the complex and overwhelming world to get our core emotional needs met.

However, as adults we certainly don't need this inner voice in the same way, and if we need it at all, there's absolutely no value in it constantly attacking and belittling us. Indeed, even when our critic gives us feedback or challenges us on something, it inevitably does it in a way that makes us feel smaller and less empowered rather than supported and motivated to make the change it's asking for.

Here's an example of what I mean. While spending time with a friend you make a joke but then immediately realize that you didn't express it in the lighthearted way you'd intended, and it could be offensive. Before you even pause to see how your friend has reacted to the joke, your inner critic immediately goes to work, attacking you, criticizing you, and making you feel like you're the worst human being ever to walk planet Earth.

In this moment, there's absolutely no opening to explore your hidden prejudice or possible unconscious privilege; instead, you're reeling from the abuse and attack of your inner critic. Unlike giving feedback to an employee in the workplace in a sensitive and skillful way, our inner critic's constant attacks give us less of what we need and want in life, not more.

Now, it's certainly true that sometimes there's a grain of truth in what our inner critic says (although often there's not). But that isn't the point. The point is that our inner critic weaponizes the grain of truth in its agenda of making us feel small and helpless. And as a result, we're less able, not more able, to act to address the grain of truth.

Our inner critic can manifest in several forms, and for some of us it's much more obvious than others. Sometimes, the more subtle the critic is, the harder it can be to spot and so the more damage it can do. Many years ago, I gave a public talk in Scotland in which I mentioned the inner critic and the impact it can have on us. Afterward, a woman came up to me and stated rather boldly, 'I don't have an inner critic. I have an inner motivator.' And yet, everything about the way she said it suggested that this motivator was far from kind and supportive – labelling itself as a force for good was just another way it avoided scrutiny and challenge.

Get RIDD of Your Inner Critic

Ultimately, to fully reset our trauma and unlock a future that isn't constrained by the sufferings of our past, we must learn to defend against and break free from our inner critic. Creating meaningful change with our inner critic can take significant effort, but I find that using a simple four-step process developed within The Diamond Approach (a path that's heavily impacted my own journey) can be immensely helpful.

In this, we need to:

1. Recognize

2. Identify

3. Defend

4. Disengage

Let's look at the four RIDD steps in detail.

1: Recognize

The first step is to recognize that we're being attacked. A huge clue that our inner critic is attacking us is feeling small and childlike or disempowered in some way. Our natural state as a human being is to feel valuable and worthy, and that our place in the world is deserved and justified, and any sign that we don't feel this way is a clue.

Just as we normalize the state of our nervous system, the same happens with our inner critic. We get so used to attacking ourselves all the time, that we normalize to being in this state, which can make it harder to recognize that, although it might feel familiar, it isn't our true, natural state.

How the Critic Shows Up

To recognize our inner critic, it's helpful to be aware that it can show up in three different ways, and we all do each of these to a varying degree:

- **Toward ourselves** – this is where we're talking to ourselves inside our own mind.

- **Projected onto others toward ourselves** – this is where we project our inner critic onto other people and imagine what they're thinking or saying about us. Effectively, we're reading others' minds and inserting our inner critic.

- **Toward others** – this is where we're judging others instead of ourselves. Often, we do this to try and inflate our own sense of worth, because of the ongoing impacts of our inner critic on ourselves.

Recognize That You're Attacking Yourself

What happens to your physical and emotional bodies when you're being attacked by your inner critic? Do you notice that you feel smaller and 'less yourself' or do you perhaps feel emotionally shut down or more defensive? Or maybe you feel a sense of hopelessness or resignation. Or is there an overwhelming feeling that everything is your fault?

Write down a few notes about what happens to you during an inner critic attack; this will help you recognize when you're attacking yourself in the future. Which of the three ways that the inner critic shows up (above) feels most familiar to you? You'll find a worksheet to help you complete this exercise in your companion course at www.alexhoward.com/trauma.

2: Identify

Once we've recognized that we're attacking ourselves, the next step is to identify the specific wording and nature of the attack. Here are some examples of inner critic attacks that you might have while reading this book:

- You're too stupid to understand what Alex is talking about.

- This might work for other people, but not for you, you're too messed up.

- You've tried changing in the past, but you never follow through.

- Exploring your emotions is just self-indulgent.

- No one else cares how you feel, so why should you?

Our inner critic will show up in every area of our lives to a degree, so really, the question isn't whether it's there in some way but how skillfully you're spotting it. Often, the content of our inner critic attacks will be shaped by the personality patterns we explored in Chapter 8. For example, if we have a strong achiever pattern, our inner critic attacks will be fueled by this and triggered by our 'failures.' Likewise, if we have a strong helper pattern, our attacks will be driven by this, and so on.

Identify Some of Your Inner Critic Attacks

Which are the most common phrases your inner critic uses when you attack yourself? Although the content of the attack might change, the types of attack it makes are fairly consistent. Write down the 10 inner critic attacks that feel the most familiar to you.

3: Defend

Once you've identified the content of your inner critic attack, the next step is to defend yourself. Having taught thousands of people over the years how to defend themselves against their inner critic, I must confess that there are two words which seem to have a somewhat sacred power and impact compared to all others: *Fuck* and *Off.*

Now, I know that for some of you using these words may feel uncomfortable. However, I find that there's a strong therapeutic value in using such colorful language. You see, because it's your inner critic that's telling you *not* to use these words, doing so is an act of defiance.

To be clear, I'm certainly not suggesting that you tell people in your life to fuck off if they criticize you (although at times it might have its place!);

the point here is that you're talking to a voice inside your mind, not a real person. It's *your* power and strength that your inner critic is using against you, and so by defending yourself against it in this way, you're taking back that power and strength.

Tell Your Inner Critic to 'Fuck Off'

As you notice your inner critic beating up on you, tell it, out loud, to *fuck off*. Then take a deep breath and become aware of how you feel. Practice doing this as often as you can. Obviously when you're around other people, it's preferable to say it inside your head, rather than out loud!

4: Disengage

When defending yourself against your inner critic, it's very important not to get into a discussion or debate about the content of the attack. With each back and forth, you're just giving your inner critic more energy and power. Therefore, once you've defended yourself against your critic, you need to shift your focus away and put it somewhere else.

It's a little like playing a game of tennis with your inner critic. You're not looking to continue hitting the ball back over the net to it in your attempts to argue and justify your value and self-worth. Instead, you're recognizing that you're being attacked, defending yourself, and then putting down your proverbial tennis racket and walking off the court.

One helpful place on which to put our focus is a positive statement we can make about ourselves. Not as an argument against what our inner critic's saying to spark more back and forth, but as something independent about ourselves that we can celebrate.

Give Positive Reinforcement

Think of 10 positive things that you recognize about yourself. They can be attributes of your character, particular skills or talents you're proud of, or things you've done in the world or for others. Now make a list of them, which you can refer to and use after you've defended. When you disengage, remind yourself of the things on this list.

So, to summarize RIDD: you're Recognizing that you're being attacked; you're Identifying the nature of the attack before Defending yourself against it; and then you're Disengaging and focusing on a positive quality or attribute about yourself. And, as with all the tools in this book, the key to success is persistent and consistent practice.

What's Possible with the Inner Critic?

While getting RIDD of your inner critic entirely is, I'm sure, a rather appealing prospect, it's not something that I've observed is realistic. What *is* possible, though, is changing our power dynamic with our inner critic and quietening its impact on us.

By constantly recognizing that we're being attacked, identifying the specific attack, defending ourselves against it, and then disengaging, over time we're fundamentally retaining this part of our mind. In so doing, it becomes much easier to be gentle and loving toward ourselves.

Let's return to Beverley's story. Growing her awareness of her inner critic was a key part of our work together. In particular, she noticed that she projected her inner critic onto other people, which resulted in her living in a world of judgement of which she was the unconscious architect. The good news was that being the architect also meant that by becoming more conscious of what was happening, she could change it.

One of the consequences of Beverley's constant barrage of projected judgement was that she was continually people pleasing and being overly accommodating of others to appease her inner critic and her imaginings of what people were thinking about her. Just as she'd learned to always put her mother's needs first, she was doing the same for everyone else in her life.

As Beverley began to defend herself against and quieten the impact of her inner critic, she learned to better boundary her relationships with others, and to listen to and ask for what she really wanted. The result was that her inner world felt easier, and her outer life of friends and relationships became more supportive and enjoyable. Beverley was also able to understand that her suffering was not her fault, but rather the product of growing up in an environment which was unable to meet her core emotional needs.

Now that we've explored the RESET model for trauma healing, it's time to look at how we can ensure that your healing isn't just in your inner world but also in your outer life with other people.

PART III

The ABCD of Trauma Healing in the Real World

INTRODUCTION

Congratulations on reaching this point in the book. We've already travelled to some challenging places, but I'm afraid I've saved the most difficult section until last. However, it's also the one with the greatest potential rewards.

For some people, a sad outcome of their journey is that although they make good progress in healing their inner world, as a direct consequence of their trauma they choose to keep themselves emotionally distanced from the outer world. Painful relationships with others are the cause of their trauma, so part of their defensive strategy is to retain the emotional walls they've built around themselves.

For me, the true measure of the impact of our healing isn't only that we find some peace and joy in ourselves – it's that despite all that we might have experienced, we've found that same peace and joy in our connection with other humans.

In fact, it's more than that: We discover that the greatest joy we can experience as humans doesn't happen in the depths of our own soul, but when our soul connects with other souls in a deep and meaningful way. When we've only known pain and suffering in our relationships with others it's hard to believe that it's through our relationships that our greatest joy can be experienced, which is why this part of our healing is so important.

It's as if there's a joy and beauty out there that we can't even imagine if we've never touched it before. And the greater our deficit in the past, the greater the wonder and beauty that can lie in our future.

To truly reset our trauma, we need to learn to let people into our hearts and lives once more. In a sense this very act is a declaration of our own transformation and healing. And so, in this final section, we're going to explore how trauma healing meets our relationships in the outside world.

I call this work the ABCD of trauma healing, which stands for:

1. Ask for help

2. Build better boundaries

3. Commit to your healing

4. Decide what your trauma means

We'll start by looking at the importance of asking for help and the power of healing in community – in a sense, this is learning to say yes to others. We'll then delve into boundaries and how to make sure you manage carefully who you invite into your inner world, which is really your capacity to say no to others.

Next, we'll move on to the importance of committing to your healing journey and how you say yes and no to yourself. Finally, we'll close with the importance of deciding what your trauma means, and how by using the tools you've learned in this book you can prevent further ECHOs in your future.

CHAPTER 15

Ask for Help
(The Power of Yes)

For some people, listening to music is a pleasant pastime, while for others, music is the language of the soul, and it makes them feel connected and alive in a way that nothing else can. I'm in the second group. In my teenage years, my discovery of angry guitar music did more to stabilize my emotional health than anything else. The impact of my musical heroes' giving words and melody to the feelings that consumed me helped me realize that I was far from alone – there were millions of others who felt the same way.

As my own trauma healing evolved over the years, the depth of my gratitude for music grew. I came to realize that for me, the theaters and arenas of live music were not just places of entertainment, there were like my church. They were where I went to feel close to myself emotionally, and to feel connected to others who felt the same way. For those few hours at a gig, I felt I was part of a community.

Music speaks to us all differently, and although I enjoy most genres, the same loud guitar music that captured my soul as a teenager still has the most precious place in my heart. And one of the bands that has especially mattered to me is Linkin Park.

In the summer of 2017, I was driving home from a family holiday and with the children traveling separately with my wife, I took advantage of the empty car by cranking up the stereo. Suddenly, a news alert came through: Chester Bennington, the lead singer of Linkin Park, had died by suicide.

I felt crushed. I'd never met Chester, but because his voice had accompanied me through some of my darkest moments, I felt as if I knew him. I'd seen Linkin Park play live a number of times in London, and the thought that I'd never again hear Chester's haunting vocals soar through an arena made me deeply sad.

Of course, as Linkin Park have sold more than 70 million albums worldwide, I wasn't alone in my grief. A few months after Chester's death, a tribute concert, featuring a who's who of rock royalty, was held at the Hollywood Bowl in LA and livestreamed on YouTube. Afterward, as there is with all grief, there was a void.

But then, something magical happened. Mike Shinoda, Linkin Park's co-vocalist and primary songwriter, went on tour himself with new material and stripped-down versions of some of the band's songs. The impact this had on the fans was profound. YouTube is full of emotional fan recordings of these concerts, and Mike speaking openly about the journey of grief.

From the moments of deep sadness to the unexpected highs of joy and celebration, and from the senseless confusion to the profound connection to the preciousness of life, these gigs allowed a healing to take place. Apart from being an excuse to share a little of my deep love of music, here's the real point I'm making: Just as our trauma doesn't happen in isolation, neither does our healing.

Coming Together with Others

When we experience trauma, often our tendency is to shut down, push the world away, and hide the wounds that we fear will never heal. Now of course we can do a huge amount to heal by using our awareness and other strategies, as you've been learning throughout this book. But there's a limit to how far this work will take us if we don't also dare to open our heart and reach out to others.

When we come together with others and let them into our heart, something magical happens. We touch and move each other in transformative ways, and in a sense, we become one big nervous system co-regulating together. And to feel the healing impact of others, we must first learn to be intimate with them. Intimacy is, in a sense, into-me-see. It's the ability to be vulnerable enough to share the depths of our pain and suffering. The more deeply we let others see into us, the more deeply we can connect and heal.

The problem is that we live in a society in which there's a great deal of cultural shame around vulnerability, showing our need for others, and dare I say it, asking for help. As I'm sure you recognize by this stage in our journey together, the point isn't whether we have emotional needs but whether we're in touch with them and working to meet them.

Put simply, there are three kinds of people in the world: 1) those who have emotional needs, are aware of them, and are open with others; 2) those who have emotional needs and are aware of them but are not open with others; and 3) those who have emotional needs but are not even aware of them. It is, of course, those in categories 2 and 3 who suffer the most.

Part of the reason why many of us who have experienced trauma push others away and prefer to be on our own, particularly when we're feeling vulnerable, is because the origins of our trauma were difficult experiences with other people. As a result, we've not only moved away from certain individuals in our lives, but we've also built walls of defense to keep others out and avoid further emotional injuries.

And yet, having the right support team around us is everything. Having the right support means we feel connected and emotionally held, and ultimately, it's depth of friendship and connection that brings our lives joy and meaning. It can take some time to build this support, so let's look at *who* can provide it and *how* we might set up these relationships.

The 'Who' and 'How' of Support

To build the support that we need in our lives, we need the right people around us, and we need the right dynamics in our interactions with them to give us (and them) the holding we want and need in a sustainable and effective way. We'll begin with the 'who' in your support circle, and then we'll focus on the 'how' of how best to set up and interact in these relationships.

Who's in Your Support Circle?

In an ideal world, our support circle would be a combination of loving family members, caring friends, and trained professionals. And right now, we might have none of these. Whatever our starting point, though, actively working to grow the circle of people who support our healing is important. And sometimes, what we need is as simple as the caring presence of humans in our physical space.

As the saying goes, we can choose our friends, but we can't choose our family. If we're lucky enough to have a loving, supportive, and emotionally sensitive family, we've truly hit the jackpot in life. For many of us, there may be elements of this, but there are likely also complexities. In the next chapter, we'll be exploring how to create appropriate boundaries when these complexities arise.

My relationships with my family members haven't always been easy, and so, particularly before I created my own family with Tania, friendships were very important. At the peak of my period of intense anxiety, which I described in Chapter 1, I felt deeply ashamed that I simply couldn't get my nervous system to relax to a safe place on my own. As I've said, this was especially the case at nighttime, when I'd lie in bed in a state of constant panic and anxiety, desperately trying to relax myself to a place of safety and peace. Previously, I'd enjoyed my own company and preferred to live alone, so I found the recognition that I needed other people around me both shameful and frustrating (thanks to my inner critic). And I also knew it to be the truth.

So, I started sharing a house with people – mostly strangers – who knew nothing of the inner turmoil with which I was living. After a few weeks I noticed it was having a profound, transformational effect. Simply having other people around with whom I could decompress at the end of the day, or perhaps watch a TV show or movie with, helped me to recalibrate my nervous system.

Once I added an effective therapist and a wider support community to the mix, I went from feeling isolated and desperately alone to beautifully supported and reminded of the healing power of simply being in the presence of other caring individuals. Human support wasn't the only factor necessary for my healing, but it was a crucial ingredient.

Forging a Heart Connection

For many of us, our friendships are more accidental than intentional. Some are event driven, in that we're pulled together around a particular project or event, and we bond in the process. Others are proximity driven and our bond is simply that they're the people who are nearest to us. Some friendships are stage driven, in that we go through a particular stage of life together and this becomes the glue of the friendship.

However, what we most want and need at the center of our friendships is a heart connection – individuals who share the same values and passions as us, who treat people with the same care that we value as important, and who, ultimately, will invite us to be vulnerable and emotionally honest.

Such connections *are* out there, but it can take deliberate time and energy to find them. As I write this final section of the book, I'm on a series of teaching weeks for our Therapeutic Coaching® practitioner training, and as each group evolves through the training, one of the additional blessings is the friendships and bonds that are being formed.

By training with people who share their passion for learning and commitment to healing, many of the participants are opening a whole new career possibility and also finding their true tribe and laying the seeds for lifelong friendships.

Be it through self-development workshops, yoga classes, meet-up groups, or the many other places where like-minded people hang out, there are few things more powerful than spending time with others on their healing journey and having a shared commitment to the potential that we all have to change and transform ourselves.

The 'How' of Support

So, now that we've talked about having the right 'who' in your life, let's turn our attention to the 'how' of these connections. Just as loving our children isn't enough on its own to become a skillful and effective parent, loving our friends isn't enough to become a skillful and effective friend. This is particularly true when it comes to offering emotional support and holding.

Those of us who have been on the receiving end of coercive and manipulative behavior in relationships, or who have been exploited for our instincts to give to and care for others, can be confused about what asking for help actually looks and feels like. And if we don't know what we're working toward, we can find ourselves allowing 'help' that just results in more pain and frustration. To help us identify the right kind of support in our life, we're going to walk through what real help is. This will also help you to offer more effective support for others in your life.

What Real HELP Looks Like

When someone gives us real help, it has four key qualities that I find work neatly into the acronym HELP:

1. Hold space

2. Express empathy

3. Listen actively

4. Positive encouragement

Let's look at the four steps of HELP.

1: Hold Space

The old saying 'A problem shared is a problem halved' might feel true in the metaphorical sense, but it shouldn't be true in the literal sense. Ultimately, the responsibility for the issues in our life lies with us. Of course, there may be times when we need practical support from others, or for a friend or loved one to help us take a very difficult step, such as reporting an incident to a person who can take action. But mostly, what we need is someone to hold space for us.

Holding space is when someone gives us a genuine invitation to be present to our emotions and feelings while we feel them. It doesn't mean that they rescue us or take over responsibility for our experience.

Some people can be very keen to take on our problems because it meets the needs of their own helper behavioral pattern, and their own self-esteem is tied to them doing so. However, healing our trauma isn't about finding other people to take it on for us – it's about growing our own resilience and capacity to meet the challenges in our lives.

The way we help each other is by providing the invitation for emotional expression – to be where we are and with what we're feeling in that moment. The real key to holding space for someone else is to stay present to ourselves. The more present to ourselves we are and connected to the moment, the more we can be present for others.

2: Express Empathy

Once someone's holding space, the next step is to express empathy. This means to witness and be sincerely interested in another person's experience. Giving a warm introduction to what we're experiencing helps us go deeper into it.

However, giving help isn't about taking on someone else's emotions. When we start overly merging with and feeling another person's emotions, our capacity to help and support them is reduced and the likelihood of us becoming emotionally drained increases.

As I said earlier, we cannot process each other's emotions and attempting to do so will leave us a lot less resourceful. Indeed, in my view, this is one of the flaws of certain counselling models – the intention that feeling the difficult feelings with the client will somehow miraculously heal them. My observation is that practitioners who work in this way end up low on energy in their own lives. In a sense they become a dumping ground for others' heaviness, when ultimately, they can't do the healing for them anyway.

Often, the thing we most need is for someone to genuinely express interest and care in our world and to invite us to come closer to ourselves emotionally. We might also be providing one another with some temporary nervous system co-regulation, but expressing empathy, done correctly, has a clear boundary between us and the other.

3: Listen Actively

Now that space is being held, and empathy is available, the next step is to listen actively. Active listening means that we're sincerely engaged in the conversation and responding with appropriate questions that help it to go deeper.

However, active listening isn't about offering solutions. Of course, it's fine if ideas spring up along the way, but imposing our own ideas on others is rarely helpful. When we go looking for emotional support and are met with rational solutions, we'll most likely feel emotionally unseen and unsupported, as well as judged and shamed.

The trick is to ask genuinely insightful and helpful questions to help guide someone toward their own answers. And when we see something on which we can give constructive feedback, to do so with permission, respect, care, and sensitivity.

4: Positive Encouragement

With space being held, empathy offered, and active listening in place, the final step is positive encouragement. This encouragement should send a message of warmth and reassurance while also coming from a grounded place. The goal isn't to try and make things better than they are, but to help the other person see the positives and the opportunities.

Remember what we talked about in Chapter 10 when we explored neuroplasticity? We train our brain by the consistent thought patterns we have, and when we find ourselves consistently in a negative frame of mind, this becomes conditioned. When someone feels actively connected to us, and we've done the previous three HELP steps, they'll be much more open to the more hopeful narrative being offered.

Do You Need More HELP?

Once you understand how HELP works, my hope is that you can recognize who is and who isn't giving you the kind of support you need; and indeed, whether you have enough such support in your life. Let's go into this further with the next exercise.

The HELP Audit

Take some time to reflect on the different areas of your life and identify where you may need more support. You might find it helpful to rate each area from 0–10, with 10 being the optimum, to help clarify where you're at right now.

Family

- How seen and accepted by your family do you feel?
- Do you feel that your family express a genuine interest in you and your life?
- How loved by your family do you feel?

Friends

- How many close friends do you have who you feel truly care about you?

- Do you spend regular time connecting with and being with your friends?

- Are you able to share your deepest experiences with your friends?

Community

- Do you feel part of an active and responsive community? This could be church, work, residents, sports clubs, children's school, and so on.

- Do you feel comfortable being yourself in your community?

- Does your community actively look out for and take care of the people within it?

Professional Support

- Do you have a therapist/coach/therapeutic professional with whom you can work through issues as needed? If not, could you consider finding one?

- Do you feel that this professional can helpfully challenge you on aspects of yourself it might be difficult to see?

- Do you feel held and cared for by someone who has no hidden agenda with you?

What do you notice after completing the HELP audit? Are there areas of your life that are rich in help and support and those where there may be room for more? It's important to remember that we all start from different places, and wherever you find yourself now is just fine. The purpose of this exercise isn't for you to start comparing yourself to others, but to have awareness of the areas you might want to work on to invite more HELP into your life.

Next Steps

I've deliberately separated the areas of life in the HELP audit as I think they all have something unique and important to give us. For example, we have a depth of history with family that we might not have with friends. And equally, professional support will offer us insight that differs from that given by those who are in a day-to-day relationship with us.

I also think it's important not to conflate some of these areas; for example, we don't want to turn our friends into our therapists or our therapist into our friend! Equally, we may not need all the people in these areas all the time. I certainly don't think that everyone should be in therapy all the time, and there may be occasions when the healthiest thing to do is to take some space from our family. Hopefully, the exercise has helped you to clarify the areas that need some focus, and your job is now to act on these.

Of course, one of the things that can be difficult to navigate when it comes to the relationships in our lives is boundaries and our ability to say no to those who aren't meeting us emotionally in the ways we need or want. This is especially true for those of us who were taught that we couldn't have boundaries, or who have people in our life who are constantly testing our boundaries. This is what we'll explore in the next chapter.

CHAPTER 16
Build Better Boundaries
(The Power of No)

One Saturday evening when I was in my mid-twenties my then girlfriend and I were relaxing on the sofa watching TV after dinner. We'd recently moved in together, and having lived alone for the previous few years, I was enjoying the comfort and familiarity of being in a fulfilling relationship. Suddenly, my mobile phone rang, and I saw that the caller was my mother. Immediately, I was concerned that something was wrong, because there was no other reason for my mother to call me so late in the day.

Within an instant of answering the phone, I realized that my mother certainly wasn't OK. She was slightly hysterical, and before she could get her words out, I'd guessed that the call would be about my sister.

My sister's mental health and behavioral issues hadn't improved since childhood, and in more recent years she'd received diagnoses of borderline personality disorder, schizoaffective disorder, and bipolar disorder. Her relationship with my mother was very destructive and abusive, and my many attempts to help unravel this – including supporting my sister and my mother separately and trying to guide and educate them toward a more functional way of relating to each other – had failed to have an impact.

A few years previously, while I was going through my therapeutic training, I'd called my sister almost daily for a year to share what I was learning. But as soon as I stopped doing the work for her, she stopped engaging. I'd realized that she liked the regular contact and energy I was giving her, but she'd no meaningful desire to change.

That evening as I sat on the sofa with my heart feeling increasingly heavy, my mother explained that my sister had become violent, smashing up part of the house, before leaving saying she was going to walk back to her home nearly 100 miles away. My mother was upset and fearful of my sister coming back, but also deeply concerned about a vulnerable person walking the streets in the middle of the night.

I had very mixed emotions. I felt empathy for my mother and concern for my sister but also deep frustration. This was the latest in a very long line of similar events, and we were stuck in a classic drama triangle in which my mother was the victim, my sister was the perpetrator, and I was the rescuer.

Always the Rescuer

Knowing what I did about psychology, I was aware of how unhealthy this situation was for all concerned. And, given that my genuine attempts to try and help the relationship between my mother and sister consistently fell on deaf ears, I found myself in an impossible situation. Effectively, my quality of life was tied to the actions of others who were stuck in a destructive dynamic with no committed action to doing anything different.

However, as I listened to my mother in her desperation, my rescuer pattern once again took over, and I told her I'd be with her as quickly as possible. On putting down the phone, I realized that it was too late to catch the last train from London, and as I didn't own a car at the time, the only option was to call a taxi. And so, I spent a small fortune on a 90-minute taxi ride, arriving at my mother's house around midnight.

My mum was still distraught and had been in touch with the police; however, busy as they were dealing with the usual Saturday night adventures, they hadn't seemed particularly interested. I decided that my first action would be to head to the local train station, which was a few miles away, and so I drove there in my mother's car. In a stroke of luck, I found my sister pacing up and down the platform, with the next train not due until 5 a.m., which was four hours away. I managed to persuade her to get in the car and then we made the two-hour journey to where she lived, which was in the opposite direction to my home.

By the time we arrived it was 3 a.m., so I slept for a few hours on my sister's sofa before driving my mother's car back to her house and then getting a train home to arrive in time for Sunday brunch. During my drive and train journey, I made some long overdue, and very difficult, decisions.

The bottom line was that being the rescuer was doing nothing to help my mother and sister, but it was doing a lot to damage my life. It wasn't that I was unwilling to give up my Saturday night to support those I loved; the problem was that this was a cycle that would never end, and my actions were likely perpetuating it.

I became increasingly aware that my endless patience and willingness to help rescue situations such as this were a stop gap that prevented things from ever becoming bad enough that more fundamental change might take place. In some ways, in my attempts to rescue them both, I was part of the problem rather than part of the solution.

Putting My Needs First

So, I decided that I needed to start prioritizing my own happiness, stability, and quality of life over being at the end of the phone for my sister's endless problems and my mother's failed attempts to fix them. Put simply, to say *yes* to myself, I was going to have to say *no* to my family.

Prioritizing my own needs didn't come easily to me, but after years of the alternative, I also knew I had no other choice. I called my mother and explained to her firmly and clearly that I was no longer available to rescue her and my sister. I loved them both, I said, but I also needed to love myself and so she should no longer call me to help in such situations.

Although it was partly fueled by a deep frustration, it wasn't an easy conversation to have. I knew that for my mother it seemed as if I was saying I didn't love her. And there were no words I could use that would make her realize that what I was doing was, ultimately, right. I also knew that my actions would leave a vulnerable person whom I loved in an even more vulnerable place. But just because doing hard things is hard, it doesn't mean we shouldn't do them.

The coming months were not an easy transition. The liberation I felt at my initial action was soon replaced by the reality of having to say no to helping in some difficult and upsetting moments. As is the case with putting any new boundary in place, I was regularly and brutally tested in my resolve. But I knew why I was doing it.

As time passed, my mother and sister continued in their dynamic, but my life did become easier. At times I found it painful and challenging to observe their suffering without doing what I could to help. And I also knew that apart from being healthy and appropriate, my actions were the only way I could truly respect and care for my own heart and emotional needs and break the cycle of drama in my life. In a sense, I was having to teach my mother and sister a new way to treat me by building better boundaries.

Healthy Versus Unhealthy Boundaries

As we discussed in Chapter 4, a boundary is a real or imagined line that indicates the limit or extent of something. A boundary separates self and other, inside and outside, and one nation and another. In the context of what we're talking about here, a boundary is our ability to stand up for what we do and don't want with others in our lives. Our boundaries can be crossed, or violated, in many ways – it might be someone standing too close to us and invading our physical or emotional space, or someone violating our time or energy by what they expect or demand of us. A boundary violation might also be the way that someone speaks to us, either in the words they use or the tone.

Creating appropriate and healthy boundaries in our relationships isn't just critical to supporting our trauma healing; it's also part of the antidote to further trauma in our future. If we don't have healthy boundaries, we're at risk of ending up in repetitive cycles of abusive relationship dynamics and finding a dysfunctional resonance with those who are looking to walk over other people's boundaries.

One of the impacts of experiencing childhood trauma is that we'll likely have grown up with unhealthy boundaries. This means we'll have normalized to dynamics and patterns with those in our life that resonate with what we know from childhood. Almost by definition, the more dysfunctional our childhood relationships, the more likely we are to find ourselves in dysfunctional relationships as adults – unless, of course, we've made a proactive and deliberate choice to move toward something different.[1,2]

It's our boundaries with others that tell them what's OK with us, and what's not. Our boundaries direct what we want more of, and what we want less of, and how it's acceptable to treat us, and how it isn't. Ultimately, healthy boundaries allow us to say yes to what we want more of, or no to what we want less of. It's our boundaries that allow us to walk toward or away from the people in our life and how they treat us.

Saying Yes to Ourselves

Learning to have healthy boundaries with others isn't just about making sure our relationships are healthy and supportive. To say yes to ourselves, we must be able to say no to other people. Put another way, to be able to make the time and space to listen to our own needs – which can be anything from focusing on our healing journey to pursuing hobbies that bring us joy – we need to be able to say no to the demands of others for our time, energy, and attention.

It might be that those demands are obvious and manageable, but for many of us they can feel relentless and overwhelming, which is all the more reason to work hard to create change in this part of our life. If we're normalized to being in toxic relationships, the chances are we almost numb ourselves to the impact of the endless demands made on us, and consequently, we neglect our own needs and wants.

While I was working hard to free myself from my own toxic relationships with family, I noticed that one of the main reasons I'd get sucked in was my tendency to be over-responsible for other people. I realized that this was particularly problematic with people who didn't take responsibility for themselves and their lives, as I'd find myself picking up the slack for them.

I remember one occasion when I was drawn into my unhealthy dynamic with my mother and sister, and I was working hard to try and support my sister to change her mood. I stepped back for a moment in total exasperation and asked myself, *whose shit is this?* In truth, the problem was with her, not me, but I was working far harder than she was to try and change it.

The Continuum of Responsibility

If we've a tendency toward a helper pattern (see Chapter 8), it makes us all the more vulnerable to finding ourselves in imbalanced relationships where we take on too much responsibility. In a sense, where there's a person who isn't taking responsibility in their life, there's an opportunity for us to step in and attempt to meet our core emotional needs by helping them.

A useful way to think about this is as a continuum of responsibility. On one end of the continuum there are people who take no responsibility at all for themselves and their life, which could also be seen as being a victim who has no ability to influence or change what's happening. On the other end, there's taking responsibility for everything and everyone, which isn't just a guaranteed recipe for stress, but also deeply unhealthy.

If you find yourself taking too much responsibility for others, it may be that you tend to allow others to manipulate you. And if you're someone who doesn't take enough responsibility, it may be that part of establishing healthier boundaries is taking more ownership of yourself and your life.

Are Your Boundaries Being Crossed?

To help us identify when we need to establish a new or stronger boundary, we must first have an early warning system for when our boundaries are being crossed. This is particularly important given how normalized we can become to the process.

A good place to start is to notice what happens in our physical and emotional bodies when our boundaries are violated. Just because we've normalized to not noticing the impact, it doesn't mean there isn't one. I know that for me, one clear sign is that my nervous system starts to activate a stress response, and another is that I feel awkward and uncomfortable, with a slightly irritated feeling.

Identify Your Response to Boundary Violations

I'd like you to take some time to explore what happens in your physical and emotional bodies when someone violates your boundaries. Which of the following signs do you notice? Remember, you can find a worksheet to help with this exercise as part of the free companion course at www.alexhoward.com/trauma.

Physical Body

- Muscular tension

- Shallow breathing

- Racing heart

- Body trying to move away

Emotional Body

- Feeling unsafe

- Shutting down emotionally

- Irritable and wanting to push away

- General feeling of discomfort

We're all different in what happens inside us when we feel that our boundaries are being crossed, so please add your own examples to this list to reflect your experience.

Identifying Gaslighting

A particularly tricky boundary violation is gaslighting – this is when someone attempts, in a coercive or manipulative way, to get us to question our own reality. The difference between gaslighting and healthy questioning is both the intention behind it and the way it's being used. As we explored earlier, sometimes there can be a grain of truth in what our inner critic says about us, but that doesn't warrant the character assassination that comes with it. The same is true of gaslighting – someone may take a small truth and use it to manipulate us into a position that's simply not true. In a sense, what they're doing is taking our core fear – that everything is our fault – and using it against us.

For example, let's say we forgot to call a loved one when we'd promised we would. There wasn't anything malicious behind it, we were simply overloaded with the other things happening in our life. But the person involved responds by weaponizing this small oversight, turning it into an entire narrative in which we're a selfish and uncaring person.

Gaslighting can have many layers and it can take some time, skill, and even professional support to fully identify it. But a good starting point is to look for the signs we've just explored around what might happen when our boundaries are crossed. A particularly strong sign that we're being gaslighted is also that we find ourselves feeling overly responsible, and something the other person has said has helped drive us toward this.

What Do Healthy Boundaries Look Like?

Now that we've examined what boundaries are, and how to know when they're being violated, let's consider what healthy boundaries look like, and how you can learn to put them in place. Establishing healthy boundaries might sound like a simple thing to do, but as any parent knows, it's often rather tricky! Healthy boundaries have some key qualities; they are...

- Strong – they're tough enough to stand up to the challenges they might face.

- Intelligent – they've been thought about and are justified and sensible.

- Loving – they feel like they're mutually respectful where possible.

- Responsive – they respond to the immediate need and can adapt to what's going to work.

- Empowering – they allow us to feel powerful and that we're worthy of standing up for ourselves.

Now, learning to put such healthy boundaries in place is a practice and it takes time. Part of this is giving yourself permission to do so and knowing that no one has the right to treat you in an unkind or manipulative way. Often, what makes it particularly difficult to follow through is our inner critic, and if that's the case for you, I encourage you to revisit Chapter 14. This may be particularly relevant when establishing healthy boundaries with parents, whose very voices are the original template for our inner critic.

Growing Your 'No'

At the heart of establishing a new boundary is being able to say no to someone. This is something we can hugely overthink, but usually the reality is far easier than the stories we tell ourselves in our head about what might happen. The key is to be calm, firm, and consistent.

If someone's speaking to us in a way that isn't respectful or isn't acceptable in our model of the world (which may well be updating as you're working through this book), then we need to tell them. Often, it may be as simple as saying, 'Please don't speak to me that way.' As it is with the inner critic, the trick is to avoid getting sucked into the detail and just holding a clear and consistent boundary.

If the person's response is to double down on their behavior and ignore your request for a boundary, that tells you some important things about them and your relationship. Indeed, it may well be a sign that you need to have more distance from this person.

Establish a Healthy Boundary

To bring this to life for you, I'd like you to put a new boundary in place in the near future.

1. Think of a person and a situation where you need a stronger boundary.

2. Spend some thinking about how you can word what you need to say in a brief, firm, and empowered way.

3. Write down your words, and practice saying them out loud in a firm and empowered way. For example, you might need to say, 'It hurts when you speak to me that way, so please stop it.' Or 'Thank you for the invitation to do xxx, but that isn't something I'd like to do at this time.'

4. The next time you see this person, practice establishing the new boundary.

Make sure you are gentle and supportive of yourself while you're putting your new boundary in place.

The Dance of Change

When you start to establish more boundaries in your life, and in doing so challenge the dynamics of your relationships, you'll likely notice that people respond in one of three ways, which I like to think of as the dance of change. Let's say that right now you're dancing the foxtrot with someone in your life, and you're in sync and step together. Then you decide you're going to dance the tango. Your partner has the following choices:

• They can come and dance the new dance with you – i.e., they can meet you in the new way of relating that you're asking for.

- They can try and pull you back into the old dance – not, perhaps, because they don't love you, but because they do, and they fear that when you change, they'll no longer be close to you in the way they're familiar with.

- You can dance separately and go your own ways.

My experience is that when we're on a proactive path of inner growth and development, we'll end up challenging many of our relationships in different ways at different points. As a result, we may find ourselves outgrowing and becoming distant from multiple people in our life.

It can feel a bit like we've cleared out all the old and outdated furniture in our house. But it takes time to fill the house with the right furniture for where we are now, and in the interim we must find peace with the emptiness and loneliness. This can be a difficult and painful part of the healing process, but if we're to change, we must be proactive.

Let the Pendulum Swing

It can also be the case that as we're figuring out what it looks, sounds, and feels like to put boundaries in place, we need to allow ourselves to go a bit too far the other way. Think of this as like a pendulum that's been held back in one direction. When it's finally released and allowed to swing, it'll go past its point of rest and balance and spend a while swinging back and forth to find that balance point.

What this might look like for you is that you've been too accommodating and too quick to ignore your own needs in relationships, but then, as you work to find a new point of balance, you find yourself saying no to certain situations which, with hindsight, you decide you didn't need to. You recognize that it was the pendulum swinging too far. But please don't worry if this happens because it's a sign of progress, and you just need some time to gradually find a new point of balance.

Of course, it isn't only other people that we need to learn to have healthy boundaries with – it's also ourselves. We're now going to turn our attention to your internal boundaries and the importance of committing to your trauma healing.

CHAPTER 17

Commit to Your Healing

Finding the right participants for my YouTube series and podcast *In Therapy with Alex Howard* isn't always easy. Of course, the first obstacle is an obvious one – it takes an enormous amount of courage for someone to be vulnerable enough to share their entire therapeutic journey on camera. However, that isn't our biggest barrier when looking for participants; indeed, since launching the series, we've been amazed by how many immensely courageous people are out there.

The real challenge is finding a sufficiently broad range of participants to reflect the wonderful diversity of modern society. With men in particular being much less likely to access therapy,[1-3] let alone talk about it, early on, we felt we could be in danger of reflecting this stereotype. Our fears were compounded when the first two men who started filming with us stopped after a few sessions. And then, in walked David.

Originally from Glasgow in Scotland, David was in his mid-forties and was suffering with debilitating depression that had resulted in regular periods of suicidal thoughts. He'd had a series of strokes during his twenties and although he'd come to terms with the impact on his mobility, it had understandably affected his confidence.

I started filming with David around nine months into the COVID-19 pandemic, and the first lockdown had hit him particularly hard. He'd lost his father a few months previously to cancer, and due to restrictions had only been able to say goodbye to him by waving through a window. He'd also lost several close friends, including one to suicide, and broken up with his long-term girlfriend. Every day, he was feeling consumed by grief and by an intense sense of hopelessness about the future.

Commitment in Action

I liked David instantly, particularly warming to his very dry Scottish sense of humor. However, I had doubts about whether he'd follow through with the therapeutic process. I knew that he wanted his life to be different, but the problem with depression is that it can sap the very energy and resourcefulness we need to invest in the process of change.

It also didn't help that a few sessions into filming with David, the UK was once more placed into lockdown, which meant he was again intensely isolated. We also had to move our sessions online. It was obvious that David was someone who didn't suffer fools gladly, and if he was going to stick with the process, he'd have to see evidence that it would be worth it.

For many years, a key part of my therapeutic approach has been to leverage my various online courses and videos to deepen patients' work outside the therapy room. After all, if someone's only spending an hour every few weeks on changing their life, it's going to have a limited impact, whereas having ongoing online resources makes a big difference.

Among the handful of people who started filming for *In Therapy* but didn't follow through, we noticed a common theme in that they had hoped the process would do the work for them and had underestimated what the process would expect from them. The process offers participants an opportunity; however, they must invest their own heart and energy into it.

As the proverb goes, 'You can lead a horse to water, but you can't make it drink.' Like I said at the start of our journey together, it's not your fault that you have trauma, but it's your responsibility to do the healing work.

To my relief, David wanted to do the work, and between our early sessions he worked through my RESET Program® in tandem with filming with me every few weeks. He did the exercises and used the tools, and things started to change for him. The changes were small at first, but in time the ripples in his life were much bigger. In a sense, a key outcome of my work with David was his learning to become his own best coach.

Learning to Self-Coach

As we near the end of our time together, I want to turn our attention to your next steps and making sure that this book isn't only an interesting read. Just as I ensured that David was doing the work outside of our sessions, I want to ensure that you do the exercises in the book and apply what you've been learning in each chapter to your life. As I said earlier, knowledge is nice, but it's action that creates change.

Of course, what's most important to prioritize and work on will be different for each person reading this, so in the spirit of any effective coach I'm going to guide you to create your own plan, as opposed to imposing a pre-defined one on you.

However, it's likely that your plan will include a meditation/mindfulness practice, working to increase your self-awareness, and applying the tools you need to drive change. To support this, we're going to focus on three key elements: the What, the How, and the What If?

By 'What' I mean what your new habits are. The 'How' relates to how you're going to approach putting them into practice – in essence, how you're relating to yourself. And 'What If' is how you'll respond if things go off track, which we can be sure at some point they will!

What Are Your New Habits?

In Chapter 10, where we talked about neuroplasticity, we explored the power of habits and how they're conditioned by whatever we do consistently. At this point, you'll have numerous daily habits and patterns that have become a normalized part of your daily routine. Some may be immensely helpful, others less so.

To reset your trauma, you don't have to change everything in your life; instead, you need to change *enough* things to tip the balance in a new direction. I think this is an important distinction to make, particularly for those of us who might have a perfectionist pattern and therefore an unobtainable image of what our healing should look like.

The good news is that what it takes to change is often not as radical as we might think in the short term. But the bad news is that it's likely to be more repetitive and tedious than we might have realized. In fact, what matters more than anything is consistency and follow-through with the daily practices and tools that work to shift our homeostatic balance to a new, healthy equilibrium.

Throughout this book, we've explored three categories of inner work. Firstly, the necessity of shifting the state of your nervous system, and the importance of tools such as meditation to help support this. Secondly, I've offered many different frameworks to help with growing your self-awareness. And finally, we've delved into specific practices to support driving change.

Having a daily meditation practice of some kind is critical. As we discussed in Chapter 9, if you need to adapt this to work with your own sensitivities, please do so. But having a practice that builds an inner sense of safety and support in your body and nervous system is key.

In almost every chapter you've completed exercises to help grow your awareness, and I strongly encourage you to revisit those multiple times, particularly as you continue working on yourself, as your responses will change and evolve over time. In a sense, self-awareness is often like peeling the layers of an onion, with each layer revealing another as our understanding deepens and expands. In terms of addressing your habits themselves, let's put something concrete in place.

Your Daily Healing Practice

To bring the work you've been doing in this book to life in the real world, I want to encourage you to commit to a daily healing practice. I suggest you spend at least 15 minutes on this, but 30–60 minutes would be ideal.

Step 1

What time of day will work best for you? For many people it's first thing in the morning, before the distractions of the day start. But if this isn't the best time for you, feel free to choose one that is. Ideally, though, a consistent time each day is best. If it's more realistic for you to commit to, say, five days a week, that's also fine.

Step 2

Start with your meditation practice (feel free to adapt the one in Chapter 9 to whatever supports you). Begin with 10 minutes and then build up to 30 minutes.

Step 3

Reflect on what's going on for you right now. You can use any of the exercises in the book, but if you need something more bespoke, work with the Therapeutic Inquiry practice in Chapter 12 to help explore what's going on for you today.

Step 4

Actively work to change your experience by using the tools in the book:

- The STOP steps – Chapter 10

- The practice of Therapeutic Inquiry – Chapter 12

- Overcoming your inner resistance – Chapter 13

- Tackling your inner critic – Chapter 14

- Asking for HELP – Chapter 15

- Putting boundaries in place – Chapter 16

What's most important here isn't getting it 'right' but getting things moving and building momentum. By establishing a daily practice that's tailored to you, you're taking an important step – not only in supporting change but doing so in a personalized way.

How Are You Supporting You?

Now that we've addressed the 'What' of your change process, we're going to explore the 'How' of your approach to it. Learning to be our own best coach and supporter isn't just a 'nice thing to have' on our healing journey – it's at the heart of navigating the often complex and twisting path of resetting our nervous system from the impacts of trauma. And, just as a great sports coach will constantly change and adapt their approach based on the needs of their athlete, the same must be true in your inner world.

In the last few chapters, we've been talking about the importance of asking for help, along with the necessity of setting and holding appropriate boundaries with others. Both skills are just as important in the inner landscape of our relationship with ourselves. Sometimes we need to give ourselves a clear and firm boundary and stop a habit or behavior that isn't helping or supporting us. Other times, we need more support and softness and to be gentler with ourselves.

When I'm training practitioners in our Therapeutic Coaching® program, I talk about this as 'pressure on' and 'pressure off' therapy. As in, when it's time to push the client harder to drive change, and equally, when they're pushing themselves too hard and things are locking up as a result, and we need to support a pressure release. Knowing which is needed and how to deliver it is part of the skill set of the therapist.

As our relationship with ourself improves, and alongside it our self-awareness, we get better at responding to our needs in a sensitive and skillful way. If you notice that your way of relating to yourself isn't as supportive and empowering as it could be, I suggest you revisit Chapter 14: Transform Your Inner Critic.

If you tend to be too hard on yourself, then learning to defend against your inner critic and soften your inner world will be important. An unfortunate effect of being too hard on ourselves is that often we become disempowered and unable to commit to following through. It's like, what's the point in trying if the story we're telling ourselves is that we're useless and bound to fail anyway?

Finding a Point of Balance

Just as a small child requires loving but firm boundaries to help shape their behavior in helpful and constructive ways, we need the same as adults, and sometimes this involves coaching ourselves to follow through with things that might not feel easy or comfortable in the short term. Just as we're learning to set boundaries for others, we're learning to do the same for ourselves in our inner world.

Self-discipline is a muscle that becomes stronger through exercise – the more consistently we commit to doing what needs to be done for us to change, the easier it'll become. And provided we do so in an intelligent and skillful way, the more we push our limits, the more they'll expand.

Indeed, that may be the very practice we need to commit to. For example, when I'm working with people with chronic illnesses, I often find they've learned that they just need to push harder; but in fact, the problem is that they're already pushing too hard, and they need to slow down, rest, and be gentler with themselves.

Remember the qualities of healthy boundaries with others we explored in the last chapter? It's those same qualities that we need to use with ourselves. Our boundaries need to be suitably strong, but they also need to be intelligent. They need to be loving and responsible, but we also need to empower ourselves.

Now, if you've spent a lifetime without healthy boundaries, it can take a while to find a place of balance. For example, if you're used to being too hard on yourself and constantly pushing, perhaps you need to go through a period of being deliberately gentle and easy with yourself.

The challenge is that you won't know what a place of balance feels like until you hit it. So, along the way, you might find yourself being too soft and not following through, and that's just fine. It's a small price to pay in your deliberate and important pursuit of more balance and having sustainable internal boundaries in your relationship with yourself.

'What If' Things Go Wrong?

Now it's time to talk about the inevitability of things going wrong! I don't say this to be negative but as the voice of reality. The hardest thing when it comes to creating change in our inner world isn't getting started – although that can be difficult – it's getting started again and again when things go off track.

Since you're reading a book about trauma, I presume that you've experienced some complex and confusing things on your life path. This means, therefore, that your healing journey probably won't be a straight line. You're going to try different things, and while some will help, others won't. This will also likely be true of elements of the approach you've been learning in this book.

The problem isn't that you'll find yourself going off track many times along the way – it's that you'll interpret being off track as failure, when in fact it's feedback. However, by going in with your eyes open, you can be prepared and ready to roll with the punches.

Furthermore, if I've learned one thing clinically from specializing in complex chronic illnesses over the last two decades, it's that often when things go off track, within the reason for them doing so is a golden nugget of information that may well help drive the next step forward.

For example, there's a common pattern we see in people who relapse on the chronic fatigue recovery journey – they try to push to do too much, too quickly and don't listen to their body. Therefore, they need to prioritize slowing down and checking in with how they feel, instead of letting their achiever pattern take over.

Furthermore, when things do go off track and we recognize they've done so – while also avoiding too much inner critic action and instead putting our energy back into the practices we've committed to – we're growing our inner discipline. In addition, if we're able to get back on track, having made some adjustments to our new plan based on what we've learned, each time we'll be taking another step closer to our ultimate goal.

And so, please go into the next stage of your healing work knowing that you'll find yourself off track many times. Being off track isn't the problem – giving up completely when you do, is. Although giving up for an hour or even a few days can be a helpful way of taking the pressure off sometimes, make sure you don't let this become your norm.

When you find yourself off track, return to this chapter and your daily healing practice (above). If you can start by coming back to the discipline of your daily exercises and tools, you'll be amazed by the impact it has.

The Rewards of Commitment

To wrap up this chapter, let's return to David's story. Developing a new way of relating to himself was critical to the lasting change he was so determined to create, and the first thing he committed to was a daily meditation practice. During meditation, he noticed some subtle but real changes in his anxiety, and a stabilization of his mood. He also realized that he couldn't meditate only when he felt like it – it had to be a daily practice. And most importantly, he needed to hold a firm boundary with himself on the days when he didn't want to meditate.

David and I also did some meaningful work on his inner critic. Again, he realized that some lively exercises with me in the therapy room wouldn't be enough, and he had to commit to continually standing up to his inner critic. And so again, he did, and it helped. As we went on to work with emotions, the same was once again true – he had to commit to embedding the new habit.

The result was that within a year, David had got himself out of a toxic living situation and had moved into a place that really felt like home. His next step was to take a different direction in his career. He found a rewarding and challenging new job, which was one of several he was offered. As things in David's life continued to improve, he didn't stop doing the practices that were helping him get there; instead, he continued to tweak and adjust them in a way that best supported him.

David's final challenge was to commit to finding a new relationship, an area that had been particularly scary for him. Over several sessions, I coaxed and challenged him to put himself out there, and with the support of the inner work he was doing, and the momentum from the changes he'd already made, he developed the courage to do so. By the end of filming, David was embarking on a new relationship for the first time in years.

As you reflect on your next steps using the principles, tools, and exercises in this book, I want you to have the same success with them as David did, because you deserve to! However, it's the actions that you commit to doing *daily* that will ultimately determine what happens. And, to show you just how powerful this work is, I'm going to finish by sharing the story of perhaps the biggest challenge I've faced in my own trauma healing.

CHAPTER 18

Decide What Your Trauma Means

I've always found driving to be a good way to relax and unwind. There's something meditative about an open road in that it requires a certain amount of focus to keep us safe but at the same time, allows us to daydream. I also like listening to loud music, and what better time to do so than while cruising along with no one around to disturb. However, on one particular car journey, my mind was far from relaxed. I had no idea what was waiting for me at my destination, but I did know *who* was waiting – my father.

A few months earlier, with the birth of our second daughter imminent, I'd said to Tania, 'I feel like a part of my soul is missing. I don't know the person that half of me has come from. I just want to have the experience of sitting in the presence of my father.'

I'd tried to find my father once before, when I was in my early twenties, but when my search hit a dead end, I'd given up. Part of me had also known that the timing wasn't right and that I wasn't ready. But now, having done a significant amount of inner work and built a stable and loving family of my own, I felt I was both strong and well supported enough to navigate whatever I'd find. And, given that my father wouldn't be a young man, I didn't have forever to wait if I wanted answers to the origins of so much of my trauma.

The Path Opens

Within a surprisingly short period of time, I'd found the address where my father was living. On the evening of my discovery, it had taken every inch of my self-restraint not to jump straight in my car and drive the couple of hours to his house.

As you can imagine, I had very mixed emotions. The little boy inside me still longed to be held by my father; the teenager in me wanted to murder him; and the young adult mostly wanted to understand why. But as I was then, more than anything, I just wanted to have the experience of sitting in his presence. Anything else would be a bonus.

Despite the intensity of my feelings, I'd done enough work in processing my hatred and rage that I no longer needed to throw it at him, and it was immensely important to me to act with grace and care, regardless of what he'd done in the past.

After speaking with a few people close to me, I decided the best next step was to ask two old friends of my parents to go to my father's home on my behalf. Neither had been in touch with him in more than 30 years, but it seemed like a softer initial approach for both of us. They would ask if he was happy to meet me, although I suspected that if he said no, I'd have gone there myself anyway. One thing I didn't feel he had the right to do was reject the little boy inside me again.

My father's old friends had traveled to where he lived, and after many hours of waiting had met him late at night, when he returned from praying at the local church. He and I had subsequently spoken on the phone for a few minutes, and the first thing he'd asked me was, 'Are you religious, son?' I'd replied that I didn't follow a formal religion, but my spiritual beliefs were very important to me. I was later to discover that he was training as a priest with the hope of working with the dying.

That day as I drove to my father's home, I reflected on our short conversation. I'd no idea how I was going to feel when I met my father, but I'd made a pact with myself – whatever happened, I was going to be true to myself. I wasn't going to shy away from difficult conversations, and if we were to have a relationship of some sort, I wanted it to be built on truth and honesty, however uncomfortable that might be.

The Gift of 'Sorry'

Before I knew it, I was parked outside my father's tiny bungalow on a council estate in the city of Canterbury, near the port of Dover in England. As I made the short walk to his front door, he came out of the house to meet me, and we hugged on the doorstep. At first, I was somewhat frozen, and the enormity of the moment didn't fully hit me. But moments later, we were sitting inside and talking.

Of course, my father had his version of events, which mostly painted him as the victim. But, given what I knew from my mum and the facts of his actions and their divorce on the grounds of his mental cruelty, I wasn't fully buying it. Clearly, he started to recognize this, and he began to change tack. Eventually, he looked at me with an expression of deep and intense regret in his eyes, and he said something that I hadn't realized I'd waited my entire life to hear: 'Son, it's not your fault. I'm sorry. I fucked up.'

As I heard the words, I started crying. Beyond everything else, soul to soul, I knew that in that moment he was sorry, and that he was owning the impact his actions had had on me. It didn't change the past, but it did soften its blows a little. After many hours of talking and spending time together, I made my way back to my own family and the loving home that Tania and I had built together.

Over the coming months, my father and I met up regularly and worked to build a relationship together. In some ways we were in a bubble of bliss and it was deeply nourishing. What was particularly moving for me was how much of myself I saw in aspects of my father. Although I recognized my kindness and loyalty as being from my mother, I clearly had my father's love of stories and interest in life's bigger questions.

A Hard Truth

However, after a while, as with all honeymoons, reality started to kick in. As much as I wanted to see the best in my father, I began to realize there was a lot more to him than met the eye. One evening, while we were having dinner in one of my favorite steak restaurants in London, I asked him in passing how his priesthood training was going. He told me he'd quit, and when I asked why, he said that they'd been too nosey, asking for background checks, and he didn't like it.

It was obvious to me that he hadn't wanted the Church to know that he'd been to prison for fraud, or that he'd gone bankrupt twice. But, to me, his refusal to disclose this was a clear sign that he was hiding from his past and quitting on something that he'd said he was passionate about. The problem was, as I said earlier, I'd made a commitment to myself that after all these years I was going to live in truth with my father. And so, I told him what I thought.

I remember my words as if I've just said them: 'The thing is, Dad, this sounds like what you did to me and my sister all those years ago. You're walking away from what you say you love because it's getting difficult.

Surely, if you have truly changed and learned from the past, you don't want to repeat the mistakes?'

Dad looked a bit taken aback by this, but the focus of the conversation soon moved on, and I thought that was it. However, as we said goodbye at Oxford Circus Underground station, heading in opposite directions, his parting words were, 'Thanks, son, for the steak, which was almost as raw as the conversation.'

When I say parting words, I mean it in the literal sense, because that was the last real conversation I ever had with my father. What had been a regular flurry of emails and phone calls stopped overnight. My father did once more what he'd done over three decades previously – he cut me off.

Doing the Work

Initially, I made excuses for the lack of contact from my father, and it took me a few months to see the reality of what was happening. But then it landed, like an atomic bomb, and I experienced a rage and hurt that no words can describe. When I say I wanted to kill him, I don't mean metaphorically – I literally wanted to kill him. For the first time in my life, I understood the force that can drive us to murder.

But, having done years of my own inner work, and as a therapist specializing in working with trauma, I knew it was now time to really put my tools to the test. Partly out of true defiance that I wasn't going to give my father the power to traumatize me again, I got to work.

Firstly, I asked for help. I worked with my therapist at the time, and I talked openly and regularly with Tania, along with several of my closest friends. But I was also very careful and selective about who I talked to; in particular, I didn't speak to those who I thought were likely to lay their own opinions on me. I needed HELP, not judgement or solutions.

In Part I of the book, we talked about the ECHOs of trauma, and how these are caused by our three core emotional needs of boundaries, safety, and love not being in place. And I worked hard to meet these needs. Firstly, I put some boundaries in place with family members whose opinions were unhelpful. Next, I committed to building safety in my nervous system using my meditation practice. Being in a loving and supportive relationship was also immensely helpful; indeed, I'd instinctively waited for this to be in place before I'd acted anyway.

It was then time to work through the RESET model. Firstly, I *recognized* what was happening. I could feel my nervous system ramping up, and my emotions shutting down and I realized this wasn't helpful. Next, I *examined* what was going on, and I could see I was going into my default achiever and helper patterns of working harder and earning validation through giving to others, in a bid to change how I felt.

I also knew there was a lot that I needed to STOP. My meditation practice was helping me to feel grounded overall, but I was also running a lot of mental patterns in the category of, 'Why has this happened to me?' and 'What did I do to deserve this?' and so I also worked hard to catch these patterns and redirect my focus and energy.

Next, it was time to work with my *emotions*. I was already fairly aware of my emotional defenses of disconnection, avoidance and distraction, and rationalizing my feelings. This allowed me to get closer to what I was *really* feeling and to inquire into my deeper truth.

I was fortunate enough to still be part of an ongoing retreat group that met twice a year (the one I talked about in Chapter 1), and I was still working with my teacher Prakash regularly. I took part in a retreat a few months later, and there's no need to guess what I worked on. I spent the week going right to the heart of my hurt, sadness, and longing, allowing myself to fully feel my rage and hatred. It certainly helped to feel validated by dear friends in the group who had known my story over many years and could truly witness me in my experience.

As part of the work, I also made sure to *transform* my inner critic and its attempts to hold a running commentary on my experience. It didn't stop my inner critic completely, but it was left with little power to affect the way I felt day-to-day. It was like a broken record playing quietly in the background, which was a nuisance, but little more.

So, what was the impact of all this? Well, it was a tough few months, and doing the work took committed effort, but on the other side of it I felt clear. I felt softer and somewhat heavy-hearted toward my father, but my hatred and rage were gone. I also felt that the little boy had grown up, and he was no longer looking to the outside to have his needs met, which was a gift in itself.

Ultimately, I felt a sense of gratitude. My primary wish had been to sit in the presence of my father, and I'd experienced that. In addition, I'd had the blessing of meeting my two much younger half-brothers, one of whom I've since become very close to. In some ways I realized that for him, growing up *with* our father in his life had been at least as damaging as my not doing so.

Put simply, it hurt, but I didn't feel that I'd been traumatized. One of the most painful things I could imagine had happened – my father had abandoned me for a second time and triggered my deepest wound. And I was able to respond in a way that meant I wasn't traumatized.

Completing My Healing

I did see my father twice more in the subsequent years, but I kept a deliberate and firm boundary. Each time, more than anything, it was to reconfirm that there was nothing I needed to say, and that I was at peace with things, which I was.

And then, almost exactly seven years after my first meeting with my father, I received news from one of my half-brothers that he'd died of a heart attack. He'd been alone when it happened, and he hadn't been found for several days. He'd also died penniless, and my parting gift to him was paying for the flowers at his funeral.

Due to COVID-19 restrictions in the UK at the time, funerals were limited to 30 people, but there were fewer than 20 people at my father's. I was grateful to have a sense of closure, and I still felt some sadness for the little boy in me; but I also felt complete in my healing. As my half-brothers spoke elegantly and lovingly of their time with our father, I found myself reflecting.

Of course, it would be unfair to compare my father's choices with my own. I hadn't lived his life, and I knew it was likely he'd had his own inner difficulties, along with some possibly undiagnosed mental health issues. And yet, I couldn't help but think about the meanings we make in life, the choices they influence, and how different my father's and mine had been.

Throughout my life, I'd made so many unconscious meanings from my father's abandonment. I'd decided that I was unlovable, that I had to take responsibility for others' feelings, and that people are not to be trusted, to name just a few.

As we saw in Chapter 6, where we talked about the outcomes of our trauma, all these meanings came with a price, and with a set of life choices as a consequence. As I've said many times now, it isn't the events of our trauma that cause us the most suffering, but what happens in our nervous system and life choices in response.

Sitting there at my father's funeral, with Tania gently squeezing my hand, I thought deeply about what I ultimately wanted my relationship with my father to mean. The answers that came to me were clear and simple: I'd lean into life when it felt difficult; I'd stand for what I believed in; and I'd love my wife and children with a ferocity and open-heartedness that nothing could destroy.

Choose an Empowering Meaning

And so, as we come to the close of our journey together, I want to ask you that same final question: What do you choose to make your trauma mean? If you don't give your trauma a meaning consciously, you'll certainly do so unconsciously, and the price you'll pay for that meaning is likely to be significant.

Ultimately, you can choose to believe that your trauma happened to you and that you're a victim. And on some level, that may well be true. But you can also choose to believe that there have been gifts and treasures you've taken from the journey that give it a different meaning.

Choosing a positive meaning for your trauma certainly doesn't mean that any perpetrators should escape appropriate justice, or that you can't have firm and powerful boundaries with them going forward. But, as one of my teachers once said to me, 'Hatred is like swallowing poison and hoping the other person dies.'

Now, to fully embody the meaning you give to your trauma, you of course need to do your healing work. If I've tried to impart one thing in this book it's that you can't bypass or ignore your emotional truth. If you have anger and hatred, let yourself feel them and digest them.

And, when all is said and done, we're left with a choice: What does it all mean? I pray that you'll choose a meaning that empowers you to live more fully, and to bring more of your gifts and potential into the world. With the global challenges we face, the world needs that from all of us now more than ever.

REFERENCES

Chapter 3: Discover Your Trauma Events

1. Felitti, V.J., et al. (1998), 'Relationship of Childhood Abuse and Household Dysfunction to Many of the Leading Causes of Death in Adults,' *American Journal of Preventive Medicine*, 14(4): 245–258.

2. Agorastos, A., et al. (2019), 'Developmental trajectories of early life stress and trauma: A narrative review on neurobiological aspects beyond stress system dysregulation,' *Frontiers in Psychiatry*, 10:118.

3. Anda, R.F., et al. (2006), 'The enduring effects of abuse and related adverse experiences in childhood: A convergence of evidence from neurobiology and epidemiology,' *European Archives of Psychiatry and Clinical Neuroscience*, 256(3): 174–186.

4. Barnes, A.J., et al. (2020), 'Identifying Adverse Childhood Experiences in Pediatrics to Prevent Chronic Health Conditions,' *Pediatric Research*, 87(2): 362–370.

5. Bellis, M.A., et al. (2019), 'Life course health consequences and associated annual costs of adverse childhood experiences across Europe and North America: a systematic review and meta-analysis,' *The Lancet. Public Health*, 4(10): 517–528.

6. Finkelhor, D., et al. (2015), 'A revised inventory of Adverse Childhood Experiences,' *Child Abuse & Neglect*, 48: 13–21.

7. Barry, T.J., et al. (2018), 'Meta-Analysis of the Association Between Autobiographical Memory Specificity and Exposure to Trauma,' *Journal of Traumatic Stress*, 31(1): 35–46.

8. Chu, J.A., et al. (1999), 'Memories of Childhood Abuse: Dissociation, Amnesia, and Corroboration,' *The American Journal of Psychiatry*, 156(5): 749–755.

9. Crane, C., et al. (2014), 'Childhood Traumatic Events and Adolescent Overgeneral Autobiographical Memory: Findings in a UK cohort,' *Journal of Behavior Therapy and Experimental Psychiatry*, 45(3): 330–338.

10. Feurer, C., et al. (2018), 'Episodic Life Stress and the Development of Overgeneral Autobiographical Memory to Positive Cues in Youth,' *Journal of Abnormal Child Psychology*, 46(8): 1563–1571.

11. Griffith, J.W., et al. (2016), 'Effects of Childhood Abuse on Overgeneral Autobiographical Memory in Current Major Depressive Disorder,' *Cognitive Therapy and Research*, 40(6): 774–782.

12. Crane, C., et al. (2014), 'Childhood Traumatic Events and Adolescent Overgeneral Autobiographical Memory: Findings in a UK cohort,' *Journal of Behavior Therapy and Experimental Psychiatry*, 45(3): 330–338.

13. Feurer, C., et al. (2018), 'Episodic Life Stress and the Development of Overgeneral Autobiographical Memory to Positive Cues in Youth,' *Journal of Abnormal Child Psychology*, 46(8): 1563–1571.

14. Griffith, J.W., et al. (2016), 'Effects of Childhood Abuse on Overgeneral Autobiographical Memory in Current Major Depressive Disorder,' *Cognitive Therapy and Research*, 40(6): 774–782.

15. Schönfeld, S. and Ehlers, A. (2017), 'Posttraumatic Stress Disorder and Autobiographical Memories in Everyday Life,' *Clinical Psychological Science*, 5(2): 325–340.

16. Sumner, J.A. (2012), 'The Mechanisms Underlying Overgeneral Autobiographical Memory: An Evaluative Review of Evidence for the CaR-FA-X model,' *Clinical Psychology Review*, 32(1): 34–48.

17. Williams, J.M.G., et al. (2007), 'Autobiographical memory specificity and emotional disorder,' *Psychological Bulletin*, 133(1): 122–148.

18. Levine, P.A. (2015), *Trauma and Memory*. Berkeley: North Atlantic Books.

19. Brewin, C.R. (2021), 'Tilting at Windmills: Why Attacks on Repression Are Misguided,' *Perspectives on Psychological Science*, 16(2): 443–453.

20. Geraerts, E., et al. (2009), 'Cognitive mechanisms underlying recovered-memory experiences of childhood sexual abuse,' *Psychological Science*, 20(1): 92–98.

21. Mcnally, R.J., and Geraerts, E. (2009), 'A New Solution to the Recovered Memory Debate,' *Perspectives on Psychological Science*, 4(2): 126–134.

22. Otgaar, H., et al. (2019), 'The Return of the Repressed: The Persistent and Problematic Claims of Long-Forgotten Trauma,' *Perspectives on Psychological Science*, 14(6): 1072–1095.

23. Herlihy, J., et al. (2002), 'Discrepancies in autobiographical memories – implications for the assessment of asylum seekers: repeated interviews study,' *BMJ*, 324(7333): 324–327.

24. Ogle, C.M., et al. (2008), 'Accuracy and Specificity of Autobiographical Memory in Childhood Trauma Victims: Developmental Considerations.' In M. L. Howe, G. S. Goodman, & D. Cicchetti (Eds.), *Stress, Trauma, and Children's Memory Development: Neurobiological, Cognitive, Clinical and Legal Perspectives*, Oxford: Oxford University Press: 171–203.

25. Ulatowska, J., and Sawicka, M. (2017), 'Recovered memories in clinical practice – a research review,' *Psychiatrica Polska*, 51(4): 609–618.

26. Chu, J.A., et al. (1999), 'Memories of Childhood Abuse: Dissociation, Amnesia, and Corroboration,' *The American Journal of Psychiatry*, 156(5): 749–755.

27. Bell, A.M., and Hellmann, J.K. (2019), 'An Integrative Framework for Understanding the Mechanisms and Multigenerational Consequences of Transgenerational Plasticity,' *Annual Review of Ecology, Evolution, and Systematics*, 50: 97–118.

28. Bridgett, D.J., et al. (2015), 'Intergenerational Transmission of Self-Regulation: A Multidisciplinary Review and Integrative Conceptual Framework,' *Psychological Bulletin*, 141(3): 602–654.

29. Dobkin, P.L., et al. (2011), 'For Whom May Participation in a Mindfulness-Based Stress Reduction Program be Contraindicated?,' *Mindfulness*, 3(1): 44–50.

30. Gapp, K., et al. (2014), 'Implication of sperm RNAs in transgenerational inheritance of the effects of early trauma in mice,' *Nature Neuroscience*, 17(5): 667–669.

31. Lê-Scherban, F. et al. (2018),' Intergenerational Associations of Parent Adverse Childhood Experiences and Child Health Outcomes,' *Pediatrics*, 141(6).

32. Short, A.K., et al. (2016), 'Elevated paternal glucocorticoid exposure alters the small noncoding RNA profile in sperm and modifies anxiety and depressive phenotypes in the offspring,' *Translational Psychiatry*, 6(6).

33. Menakem, R. (2021), *My Grandmother's Hands: Racialized Trauma and the Pathway to Mending Our Hearts and Bodies*. London: Penguin Books Ltd.

34. Wolynn, M. (2022), *It Didn't Start With You*. London: Vermilion.

35. Hübl, T. (2020), *Healing Collective Trauma: A Process for Integrating Our Intergenerational and Cultural Wounds*, Louisville: Sounds True.

Chapter 4: Context Is Everything

1. Ciaunica, A., et al. (2021), 'The "First Prior": from Co-Embodiment to Co-Homeostasis in Early Life,' *Consciousness and Cognition*, 91.

2. Graf, N., et al. (2022), 'Neurobiology of Parental Regulation of the Infant and Its Disruption by Trauma Within Attachment,' *Frontiers in Behavioral Neuroscience*, 16.

3. Porges, S.W. (2022), 'Polyvagal Theory: A Science of Safety,' *Frontiers in Integrative Neuroscience*, 16.

4. Townshend, K., and Caltabiano, N.J. (2019), 'The extended nervous system: affect regulation, somatic and social change processes associated with mindful parenting,' *BMC Psychology*, 7(1).

5. Azhari, A., et al, (2019), 'Parenting Stress Undermines Mother-Child Brain-to-Brain Synchrony: A Hyperscanning Study,' *Scientific Reports*, 9(1).

6. Esposito, G., et al. (2017), 'Response to Infant Cry in Clinically Depressed and Non-Depressed Mothers,' *PLoS ONE*, 12(1).

7. Ostlund, B.D., et al. (2017), 'Shaping emotion regulation: attunement, symptomatology, and stress recovery within mother–infant dyads,' *Developmental Psychobiology*, 59(1): 15–25.

8. Saxbe, D., et al. (2015), 'Neural correlates of parent–child HPA axis coregulation,' *Hormones and Behavior*, 75: 25–32.

9. Viaux-Savelon, S., et al. (2022), 'Infant Social Withdrawal Behavior: A Key for Adaptation in the Face of Relational Adversity,' *Frontiers in Psychology*, 13.

10. Hambrick, E.P., et al. (2019), 'Timing of Early-Life Stress and the Development of Brain-Related Capacities,' *Frontiers in Behavioral Neuroscience*, 13.

11. Kumsta, R., et al. (2017), 'HPA axis dysregulation in adult adoptees twenty years after severe institutional deprivation in childhood,' *Psychoneuroendocrinology*, 86: 196–202.

12. Strathearn, L., et al. (2020), 'Long-term Cognitive, Psychological, and Health Outcomes Associated with Child Abuse and Neglect,' *Pediatrics*, 146(4).

13. Widom, C.S., et al. (2012), 'A prospective investigation of physical health outcomes in abused and neglected children: New findings from a 30-year follow-up.' *American Journal of Public Health*, 102(6): 1135–1144.

14. Beijers, R., et al. (2016), 'An experimental study on mother-infant skin-to-skin contact in full-terms,' *Infant Behavior & Development*, 43: 58–65.

15. Cascio, C.J., et al. (2019), 'Social touch and human development,' *Developmental Cognitive Neuroscience*, 35: 5–11.

16. Cooijmans, K.H.M., et al. (2022), 'Daily mother-infant skin-to-skin contact and maternal mental health and postpartum healing: a randomized controlled trial,' *Scientific Reports*, 12(1).

17. Fotopoulou, A., et al. (2022), 'Affective regulation through touch: homeostatic and allostatic mechanisms,' *Current Opinion in Behavioral Sciences*, 43: 80–87.

18. Morrison, I. (2016), 'Keep Calm and Cuddle on: Social Touch as a Stress Buffer,' *Adaptive Human Behavior and Physiology*, 2(4), 344–362.

19. Narvaez, D., et al. (2019), 'The importance of early life touch for psychosocial and moral development,' *Psicologia, Reflexão e Crítica: Revista Semestral Do Departamento de Psicologia Da UFRGS*, 32(1).

Chapter 5: How's Your Homeostatic Balance?

1. Godoy, L.D., et al. (2018), 'A comprehensive overview on stress neurobiology: Basic concepts and clinical implications,' *Frontiers in Behavioral Neuroscience*, 12, 127.

2. Maté, G. (2019) *When the Body Says No: The Cost of Hidden Stress.* London: Vermilion.

3. Kinlein, S.A., et al. (2015), 'Dysregulated hypothalamic-pituitary-adrenal axis function contributes to altered endocrine and neurobehavioral responses to acute stress,' *Frontiers in Psychiatry*, 6: 31.

4. Porges, S.W. (2022), 'Polyvagal Theory: A Science of Safety,' *Frontiers in Integrative Neuroscience*, 16.

5. Godbout, J.P. and Glaser, R. (2006), 'Stress-Induced Immune Dysregulation: Implications for Wound Healing, Infectious Disease and Cancer,' *Journal of Neuroimmune Pharmacology*, 1(4): 421–427.

6. Heim, C., et al. (2009), 'Childhood trauma and risk for chronic fatigue syndrome: association with neuroendocrine dysfunction,' *Archives of General Psychiatry*, 66(1): 72–80.

7. Kolacz, J. and Porges, S.W. (2018), 'Chronic Diffuse Pain and Functional Gastrointestinal Disorders After Traumatic Stress: Pathophysiology Through a Polyvagal Perspective,' *Frontiers in Medicine*, 5: 145.

8. McManus, E., et al. (2021), 'The Effects of Stress Across the Lifespan on the Brain, Cognition and Mental Health: A UK Biobank study,' *Neurobiology of Stress*, 18.

9. Morris, G. and Maes, M. (2014), 'Oxidative and Nitrosative Stress and Immune-Inflammatory Pathways in Patients with Myalgic Encephalomyelitis (ME)/Chronic Fatigue Syndrome (CFS),' *Current Neuropharmacology*, 12(2): 168–185.

10. Schakel, L., et al. (2019), 'Effectiveness of Stress-Reducing Interventions on the Response to Challenges to the Immune System: A Meta-Analytic Review,' *Psychotherapy and Psychosomatics*, 88(5): 274–286.

11. Duan, H., et al. (2013), 'Chronic stress exposure decreases the cortisol awakening response in healthy young men,' *Stress: The International Journal on the Biology of Stress*, 16(6): 630–637.

12. Russell, A.L., et al. (2018), 'Factors promoting vulnerability to dysregulated stress reactivity and stress-related disease,' *Journal of Neuroendocrinology*, 30(10).

13. Gerritsen, L., et al. (2017), 'HPA Axis Genes, and Their Interaction with Childhood Maltreatment, are Related to Cortisol Levels and Stress-Related Phenotypes,' *Neuropsychopharmacology*, 42(12): 2446–2455.

14. Kempke, S., et al. (2015), 'Effects of Early Childhood Trauma on Hypothalamic-Pituitary-Adrenal (HPA) Axis Function in Patients with Chronic Fatigue Syndrome,' *Psychoneuroendocrinology*, 52: 14–21.

15. Kumsta, R., et al. (2017), 'HPA axis dysregulation in adult adoptees twenty years after severe institutional deprivation in childhood,' *Psychoneuroendocrinology*, 86: 196–202.

16. Shalev, I., et al. (2020), 'Investigating the impact of early-life adversity on physiological, immune, and gene expression responses to acute stress: A pilot feasibility study,' *PLoS ONE*, 15(4).

17. Afari, N., et al. (2014), 'Psychological Trauma and Functional Somatic Syndromes: A Systematic Review and Meta-Analysis,' *Psychosomatic Medicine*, 76(1), 2–11.

18. Godbout, J.P. and Glaser, R. (2006), 'Stress-Induced Immune Dysregulation: Implications for Wound Healing, Infectious Disease and Cancer,' *Journal of Neuroimmune Pharmacology*, 1(4): 421–427.

19. Morris, G., et al. (2019), 'Myalgic encephalomyelitis or chronic fatigue syndrome: how could the illness develop?' *Metabolic Brain Disease*, 34(2): 385–415.

20. Naviaux, R.K. (2014), 'Metabolic features of the cell danger response,' *Mitochondrion*, 16: 7–17.

Chapter 6: The Outcomes of Your Trauma

1. Cosgrove, L. and Wheeler, E.E. (2013), 'Industry's colonization of psychiatry: Ethical and practical implications of financial conflicts of interest in the DSM-5,' 23(1): 93–106.

2. Frances, A. (2013), 'The New Crisis in Confidence in Psychiatric Diagnosis,' *Annals of Internal Medicine*, 159(3): 221–222.

3. Bredström, A. (2017), 'Culture and Context in Mental Health Diagnosing: Scrutinizing the DSM-5 Revision,' *Journal of Medical Humanities*, 40(3): 347–363.

4. Ussher, J.M. (2013), 'Diagnosing difficult women and pathologising femininity: Gender bias in psychiatric nosology,' *Feminism and Psychology*, 23(1): 63–69.

5. Davies, J. (2014). *Cracked: Why Psychiatry is Doing More Harm than Good.* London: Icon Books.

6. Achenbach, J., et al. (2019), 'Childhood traumatization is associated with differences in TRPA1 promoter methylation in female patients with multisomatoform disorder with pain as the leading bodily symptom,' *Clinical Epigenetics*, 11(1).

7. Brown, R.C., et al. (2018), 'Associations of adverse childhood experiences and bullying on physical pain in the general population of Germany,' *Journal of Pain Research*, 11: 3099–3108.

8. Kascakova, N., et al. (2020), 'The Unholy Trinity: Childhood Trauma, Adulthood Anxiety, and Long-Term Pain,' *International Journal of Environmental Research and Public Health*, 17(2).

9. Kolacz, J. and Porges, S.W. (2018), 'Chronic Diffuse Pain and Functional Gastrointestinal Disorders After Traumatic Stress: Pathophysiology Through a Polyvagal Perspective.' *Frontiers in Medicine*, 5, 145.

10. Yeung, E.W., et al. (2016), 'Cortisol Profile Mediates the Relation between Childhood Neglect and Pain and Emotional Symptoms among Patients with Fibromyalgia,' *Annals of Behavioral Medicine*, 50(1): 87–97.

11. Lipton, B. (2016), *The Biology Of Belief*. London: Hay House.

12. Cowan, N. (2001), 'The magical number 4 in short-term memory: a reconsideration of mental storage capacity,' *The Behavioral and Brain Sciences*, 24(1): 87–114.

13. Cowan, N. (2015), 'George Miller's Magical Number of Immediate Memory in Retrospect: Observations on the Faltering Progression of Science.' *Psychological Review*, 122(3): 536–541.

14. Encyclopedia Britannica, 'Information theory,' www.britannica.com/science/information-theory/Physiology [Accessed August 30, 2022]

15. Hilbert, M. (2012), 'Toward a synthesis of cognitive biases: how noisy information processing can bias human decision making,' *Psychological Bulletin*, 138(2): 211–237.

16. Lieder, F., et al. (2018), 'Over-representation of extreme events in decision-making reflects rational use of cognitive resources,' *Psychological Review*, 125(1): 1–32.

17. Santos, L.R. and Rosati, A.G. (2015), 'The Evolutionary Roots of Human Decision Making,' *Annual Review of Psychology*, 66: 321–347.

Chapter 7: Recognize Which State Your Nervous System Is In

1. Van der Kolk, B. (2015), *The Body Keeps the Score*. London: Penguin Books Ltd.

Chapter 9: Stop Running, Start Feeling

1. Bridgett, D.J., et al. (2015), 'Intergenerational Transmission of Self-Regulation: A Multidisciplinary Review and Integrative Conceptual Framework,' *Psychological Bulletin*, 141(3): 602–654.

2. Townshend, K. and Caltabiano, N.J. (2019), 'The extended nervous system: affect regulation, somatic and social change processes associated with mindful parenting,' *BMC Psychology*, 7(1).

3. Graf, N., et al. (2022), 'Neurobiology of Parental Regulation of the Infant and Its Disruption by Trauma Within Attachment,' *Frontiers in Behavioral Neuroscience*, 16.

4. Saxbe, D., et al. (2015), 'Neural correlates of parent–child HPA axis coregulation,' *Hormones and Behavior*, 75: 25–32.

5. Vink, M., et al. (2020), 'Towards an integrated account of the development of self-regulation from a neurocognitive perspective: A framework for current and future longitudinal multi-modal investigations,' *Developmental Cognitive Neuroscience*, 45.

6. Azhari, A., et al. (2019), 'Parenting Stress Undermines Mother-Child Brain-to-Brain Synchrony: A Hyperscanning Study,' *Scientific Reports*, 9(1).

7. Cashman, K.D. (2007), 'Vitamin D in childhood and adolescence,' *Postgraduate Medical Journal*, 83(978): 230–235.

8. Esposito, G., et al. (2017), 'Response to Infant Cry in Clinically Depressed and Non-Depressed Mothers,' *PLoS ONE*, 12(1).

9. Kumsta, R., et al. (2017), 'HPA axis dysregulation in adult adoptees twenty years after severe institutional deprivation in childhood,' *Psychoneuroendocrinology*, 86: 196–202.

10. Ostlund, B.D., et al. (2017), 'Shaping emotion regulation: attunement, symptomatology, and stress recovery within mother–infant dyads,' *Developmental Psychobiology*, 59(1): 15–25.

11. Sanders, M.R. and Hall, S. L. (2018), 'Trauma-informed care in the newborn intensive care unit: promoting safety, security and connectedness,' *Journal of Perinatology*, 38(1): 3–10.

12. Black, D.S. and Slavich, G.M. (2016), 'Mindfulness meditation and the immune system: a systematic review of randomized controlled trials,' *Annals of the New York Academy of Sciences*, 1373(1): 13–24.

13. Creswell, J.D., et al. (2019), 'Mindfulness Training and Physical Health: Mechanisms and Outcomes,' *Psychosomatic Medicine*, 81(3): 224–232.

14. Pascoe, M.C., et al. (2021), 'Psychobiological mechanisms underlying the mood benefits of meditation: A narrative review,' *Comprehensive Psychoneuroendocrinology*, 6.

15. Schlechta Portella, C.F., et al. (2021), 'Meditation: Evidence Map of Systematic Reviews,' *Frontiers in Public Health*, 9.

16. Zhang, D., et al. (2021), 'Mindfulness-based interventions: an overall review,' *British Medical Bulletin*, 138(1): 41–57.

17. Zhu, L., et al. (2021), 'Mind–Body Exercises for PTSD Symptoms, Depression, and Anxiety in Patients With PTSD: A Systematic Review and Meta-Analysis,' *Frontiers in Psychology*, 12.

18. Burrows, L. (2015), 'Safeguarding Mindfulness Meditation for Vulnerable College Students,' *Mindfulness*, 7(1): 284–285.

19. Dobkin, P.L., et al. (2011), 'For Whom May Participation in a Mindfulness-Based Stress Reduction Program be Contraindicated? *Mindfulness*, 3(1): 44–50.

20. Zhu, J., et al. (2019), 'Trauma- and Stressor-Related History and Symptoms Predict Distress Experienced during a Brief Mindfulness Meditation Sitting: Moving toward Trauma-Informed Care in Mindfulness-Based Therapy,' *Mindfulness*, 10(10): 1985–1996.

21. Kelly, A. and Garland, E.L. (2016), 'Trauma-Informed Mindfulness-Based Stress Reduction for Female Survivors of Interpersonal Violence: Results From a Stage I RCT,' *Journal of Clinical Psychology*, 72(4): 311–328.

22. Chen, L., et al. (2015), 'Eye movement desensitization and reprocessing versus cognitive-behavioral therapy for adult posttraumatic stress disorder: systematic review and meta-analysis,' *The Journal of Nervous and Mental Disease*, 203(6): 443–451.

23. Church, D., et al. (2018), 'Guidelines for the Treatment of PTSD Using Clinical EFT (Emotional Freedom Techniques),' *Healthcare*, 6(4).

24. Khan, A.M., et al. (2018), 'Cognitive Behavioral Therapy versus Eye Movement Desensitization and Reprocessing in Patients with Post-traumatic Stress Disorder: Systematic Review and Meta-analysis of Randomized Clinical Trials,' *Cureus*, 10(9).

Chapter 10: Put a STOP to Your Unhelpful Behaviors

1. Albert, P.R. (2019), 'Adult neuroplasticity: A new "cure" for major depression?' *Journal of Psychiatry & Neuroscience*, 44(3): 147–150.

2. Phillips, C. (2017), 'Lifestyle Modulators of Neuroplasticity: How Physical Activity, Mental Engagement, and Diet Promote Cognitive Health during Aging,' *Neural Plasticity*, vol. 2017.

3. Bartol, T.M., et al. (2015),' Nanoconnectomic upper bound on the variability of synaptic plasticity,' *eLife*, 4.

Chapter 16: Build Better Boundaries (the Power of No)

1. Johnson, S. (2011), *Hold Me Tight*. London: Piatkus

2. Wolynn, M. (2022), *It Didn't Start With You*. London: Vermilion.

Chapter 17: Commit to Your Healing

1. Fleury, M.J., et al. (2014), 'Determinants and patterns of service utilization and recourse to professionals for mental health reasons,' *BMC Health Services Research*, 14(1).

2. Gonzalez, J.M., et al. (2005), 'How do attitudes toward mental health treatment vary by age, gender, and ethnicity/race in young adults?,' *Journal of Community Psychology*, 33(5): 611–629.

3. Nam, S.K., et al. (2010), 'A Meta-analysis of Gender Differences in Attitudes Toward Seeking Professional Psychological Help,' *Journal of American College Health*, 59(2): 110–116.

ACKNOWLEDGMENTS

The hardest part of writing this book wasn't the writing process itself – it was the many years of personal struggle and living the material in my own life to truly understand it. The list of people who impacted or influenced me along that journey is immense and would fill a book of its own, so, to those of you I practiced with, inquired with, laughed with, cried with, and learned with, thank you from the bottom of my heart.

This book also wouldn't have been possible without the incredible work of the 80+ team members across the various businesses within the Alex Howard Group. From the practitioner teams in The Optimum Health Clinic, to the production teams in Conscious Life, and everyone in between, it's your commitment to excellence that inspires me every day and helps me to grow and refine my own understandings, many of which have found their way into this book.

In particular, I want to acknowledge my dear friend Anna Duschinsky, not only for her friendship but for helping me shape and develop the Therapeutic Coaching® model over the last 20 years. Teaching together on our practitioner training residentials is always a highlight of my year.

I also want to thank my core support team of Anna Kittow, Grace Allen, and Gemma Dent who help keep the core pillars of the organization flourishing day-to-day, and who put up with my endless rambling voice memos, always responding to them with a smile and a can-do attitude!

Thank you to my commissioning editor at Hay House, Helen Rochester, for believing so fully in the book, and for not letting me off the hook until we got the right title, regardless of the extra work it kept making for all of us! Huge thanks to my editor, Debra Wolter, for her patient and diligent work in knocking my writing into shape – you make me sound like me, only better!

Huge appreciation also to Sarah Benjamins, my researcher, who painstakingly went through my various drafts to make sure I was fairly representing the science and made some excellent suggestions along the way to strengthen my positions. Sorry for all the late nights!

Finally, thank you to my endlessly patient wife Tania. Much of the clarity of my thinking comes from our reflections on how we can attempt to break the cycles of trauma with our daughters, Marli, Ariella, and Lyra. We certainly don't always get it right, but I hope that the depth of our attempts is a sign of how deeply we love you girls.

INDEX

Exercises are given in *italics*

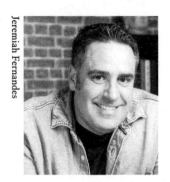

Jeremiah Fernandes

ABOUT THE AUTHOR

Alex Howard is the CEO of the Alex Howard Group, an international group of businesses which includes The Optimum Health Clinic, online learning platform Conscious Life, online coaching program the RESET Program®, and professional training programs Therapeutic Coaching® and Therapeutic Nutrition.

Alex is passionate about making physical and emotional healing accessible to everyone, and in the last few years his online Super Conference series has been attended by more than 1 million people. Alex has also published academic research in journals including *British Medical Journal Open* and *Psychology & Health* and is the author of the books *Why Me?* and *Decode Your Fatigue.* Since March 2020, he has been documenting his therapeutic work with real-life patients via his *In Therapy with Alex Howard* YouTube series.

www.alexhoward.com

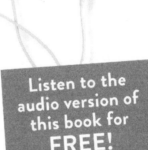

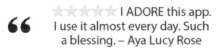

HAY HOUSE
Online Video Courses

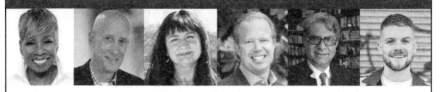

Your journey to a better life starts with figuring out which path is best for you. Hay House Online Courses provide guidance in mental and physical health, personal finance, telling your unique story, and so much more!

LEARN HOW TO:

- choose your words and actions wisely so you can tap into life's magic
- clear the energy in yourself and your environments for improved clarity, peace, and joy
- forgive, visualize, and trust in order to create a life of authenticity and abundance
- manifest lifelong health by improving nutrition, reducing stress, improving sleep, and more
- create your own unique angelic communication toolkit to help you to receive clear messages for yourself and others
- use the creative power of the quantum realm to create health and well-being

To find the guide for your journey,
visit www.HayHouseU.com.

HAY HOUSE
online learning

HAY
HOUSE

CONNECT WITH

HAY HOUSE
ONLINE

🌐 hayhouse.co.uk   f @hayhouse

📷 @hayhouseuk   🐦 @hayhouseuk

▶ @hayhouseuk   ♪ @hayhouseuk

Find out all about our latest books & card decks • Be the first to know about exclusive discounts • Interact with our authors in live broadcasts • Celebrate the cycle of the seasons with us • Watch free videos from your favourite authors • Connect with like-minded souls

'The gateways to wisdom and knowledge
are always open.'

Louise Hay